SELF-ASSESSMENT OF CURRENT KNOWLEDGE IN PSYCHIATRY

By

PAUL SALKIN, M.D.

1200 MULTIPLE CHOICE QUESTIONS AND REFERENCED ANSWERS

MEDICAL EXAMINATION PUBLISHING COMPANY, INC.

65-36 Fresh Meadow Lane

Flushing, N.Y. 11365

1972

Library of Congress
Catalog Card Number
78-160718

ISBN   0-87488-252-4

June 1972

SELF-ASSESSMENT OF CURRENT KNOWLEDGE

IN PSYCHIATRY

TABLE OF CONTENTS

PREFACE

This book consists of questions derived from articles in recent journals of psychiatry. It is offered as an aid in self-assessment of current knowledge for psychiatrists, and it will also be useful to medical students, psychiatric residents, and those preparing for licensure and Board examinations.

The questions are presented in various forms so that the reader will become familiar with current examination methods, and an answer key is provided. Each question is referenced to the specific article of its source, and it is important that the articles be consulted so that the reader can obtain a broader and more substantial base of knowledge.

Paul Salkin, M.D.

FOR EACH MULTIPLE CHOICE QUESTION, SELECT THE MOST
APPROPRIATE COMPLETION:

1. CONTINGENT NEGATIVE VARIATION (CNV) IS A SHIFT IN THE EEG
    BASELINE THAT:
    A. Is seen when the subject is probably dreaming
    B. Occurs in the deepest stage of sleep
    C. Depends on the association of two successive stimuli
    D. Is seen during depression   Ref. 1 - p. 1

2. CNV HAS A CONSISTENT RELATIONSHIP TO:
    A. Expectancy, conation, and attention
    B. Affective states
    C. Seizure disorders
    D. Dream content
    E. Dream deprivation   Ref. 1 - p. 1

3. GREY WALTER HAS CONCLUDED THAT USING CNV AS A CRITERION:
    A. It seems reasonable to accept the age 21 as the beginning of the years
       of discretion
    B. One may be able to predict mood swings
    C. Intelligence can be assessed
    D. Dreams are likely to be occurring
    E. The stage of sleep can be determined
                                          Ref. 1 - p. 8

4. CNV REFLECTS SLOW ELECTRICAL ACTIVITY IN LARGE AREAS OF
    THE:
    A. Occipital lobes
    B. Parietal lobes
    C. Temporal lobes
    D. Frontal lobes
    E. Thalamus   Ref. 1 - p. 13

5. PHENOBARBITAL, REDUCED BY 30 MG/DAY, MAY BE USED IN
    WITHDRAWAL FROM:
    A. Addiction to both long-acting and short-acting barbiturates
    B. Glutethimide addiction
    C. Meprobamate addiction
    D. All of the above
    E. None of the above   Ref. 2 - pp. 57-58

6. A SIGNIFICANT FACTOR IN BEHAVIOR THERAPY IS:
    A. History taking
    B. Transference
    C. Suggestion
    D. All of the above
    E. None of the above   Ref. 3 - pp. 22-28

7. A DRUG THAT HAS RECENTLY BEEN FOUND EFFECTIVE IN PAR-
    KINSON'S DISEASE IS:
    A. DOM
    B. DOET
    C. L-asparaginase
    D. Poly I:C
    E. L-DOPA   Ref. 4 - p. 61

6

8. THIS TREATMENT FOR PARKINSON'S DISEASE WAS DEVELOPED BY:
   A. Kline
   B. Cotzias
   C. Hofmann
   D. Delay
   E. Pitnam
   Ref. 4 - p. 61

9. SIDE EFFECTS OF THIS TREATMENT FREQUENTLY NOTED INCLUDE:
   A. Narcolepsy
   B. Spontaneous penile erection
   C. Retinitis pigmentosa
   D. Glycosuria
   E. Convulsions
   Ref. 4 - p. 64

10. THE CATECHOLAMINE (CA) HYPOTHESIS OF MOOD STATES THAT:
    A. Some depressions are associated with deficiency of CA at CNS sites
    B. Some depressions are associated with increase of CA at CNS sites
    C. Increased CA causes depression
    D. Decreased CA causes depression
    E. None of the above
    Ref. 5 - p. 68

11. RECENT STUDIES, CONTRARY TO WHAT WOULD BE PREDICTED BY THE CATECHOLAMINE HYPOTHESIS OF MOOD, HAVE DEMONSTRATED THAT:
    A. Plasma CA concentration was decreased in depression
    B. Plasma CA concentration was increased in depression
    C. Plasma CA cannot be measured accurately
    D. Anxiety has no effect on urinary excretion of CA
    E. None of the above
    Ref. 5 - p. 68

12. AN IMPAIRMENT COMMON TO CHRONIC ALCOHOLICS IS:
    A. Amblyopia
    B. Disturbance of performance on sensory-motor tests
    C. Scanning speech
    D. Cog-wheel rigidity
    E. Diminished abstracting ability
    Ref. 6 - p. 74

13. THE ABOVE IMPAIRMENT SUGGESTS BRAIN DAMAGE IN SEVERAL AREAS, BUT NOT IN THE:
    A. Dorsolateral aspects of frontal lobes
    B. Motor strip of the frontal lobes
    C. Hypothalamus
    D. Thalamus
    E. Wall of the third ventricle and aqueduct
    Ref. 6 - p. 74

14. HALLUCINATIONS ARE COMMON IN WHICH OF THE FOLLOWING DISORDERS?:
    A. Affective disorders
    B. Chronic schizophrenia
    C. Acute schizophrenia
    D. Organic brain syndrome
    E. All of the above
    Ref. 7 - p. 77

15. A TYPE OF HALLUCINATION MORE CHARACTERISTIC OF AN ACUTE
CONDITION IS:
A. Auditory
B. Visual
C. Gustatory
D. Tactile
E. Olfactory   Ref. 7 - p. 79

16. THE MOST COMMON FORM OF HALLUCINATION IS:
A. Auditory
B. Visual
C. Tactile
D. Olfactory
E. Gustatory   Ref. 7 - p. 78

17. VISUAL HALLUCINATIONS:
A. Are usually experienced in color
B. Most often occur in organic brain syndromes and alcoholism
C. Are usually of normal-sized, normal-appearing persons
D. Of animals occur most often in alcoholism
E. All of the above   Ref. 7 - p. 78

18. HALLUCINATIONS MAY OCCUR:
A. In hysteria
B. When alcohol is withdrawn from alcoholics
C. In the form of derogatory voices in schizophrenia
D. All of the above
E. None of the above   Ref. 7 - p. 76

19. A REVIEW OF THE 26 CONTROLLED DOUBLE-BLIND STUDIES OF THE
EFFICACY OF MEPROBAMATE IN RELIEVING ANXIETY REVEALED
THAT:
A. None of the studies demonstrated it to be more effective than placebo
B. Five of the studies demonstrated it to be more effective than placebo
C. Twenty of the studies demonstrated it to be more effective than placebo
D. All such studies have demonstrated its superior effectiveness
E. No such studies have been performed to date
                                       Ref. 8 - p. 1299

20. SIGNIFICANT FACTORS CONTRIBUTING TO WIDESPREAD USE OF A
DRUG INCLUDE:
A. Clinical effectiveness
B. Reports in the news media
C. Advertisements and appealing brand name
D. All of the above
E. None of the above   Ref. 8 - p. 1298

21. THE MOST CONSISTENT FINDING REPORTED IN PSYCHIATRIC
EPIDEMIOLOGY STUDIES IS:
A. An inverse relation between disorder and social class
B. A progressive decrease in the rate of suicide
C. That too early hospital discharge causes no complications
D. That the prevalence of mental disorder is lower than would have been
expected
E. A decline in the incidence of mental disorder
                                       Ref. 9 - p. 1307

22. BUEHLER'S "DEPRESSIVE EFFECT" OCCURS:
    A. Following the use of chlorpromazine and other phenothiazines
    B. During the course of infectious and serum hepatitis
    C. During the review of psychiatric interview records
    D. In deprived infants
    E. When there is mother-infant separation in monkeys
    Ref. 9 - p. 1313

23. THE A-D CASENESS RATING SCALE:
    A. Was used in the Midtown Study but not in the Stirling County Study
    B. Is used to estimate the severity of illness
    C. Is used to estimate the probability of being a case
    D. Can be used in the differential between neurosis and psychosis
    E. Is not suitable in psychiatric epidemiology
    Ref. 9 - p. 1312

24. IN THE EPIDEMIOLOGICAL INVESTIGATION OF PREVALENCE OF
    MENTAL DISORDER:
    A. Interviewers tend to rate subjects as more impaired than do reviewers
       of written records of interviews
    B. Class bias is no longer a factor operating in clinical judgment
    C. Collection procedures may differ but results tend to be uniform
    D. Psychiatric interviewers see something in individuals that reviewers
       of recorded data overlook
    E. Community leaders show a lower rate of mental illness on the reviewer
       Psychiatric Status Schedule (PSS)   Ref. 9 - p. 1307

25. THE THIRD STAGE IN THE CHILD'S REACTION TO SEPARATION FROM
    THE MOTHER:
    A. Has been frequently duplicated in the infant monkey
    B. Is called the stage of detachment (Bowlby)
    C. Leads to a symbiotic psychosis (Mahler)
    D. Is the stage of protest
    E. Is amenable to treatment with imipramine
    Ref. 10 - p. 1314

26. INFANT MONKEYS SEPARATED FROM THEIR MOTHERS:
    A. React with an initial stage of protest
    B. Usually show no reaction
    C. Usually demonstrate a stage of detachment
    D. React with behavior strikingly different from that of human infants
    E. React with silence   Ref. 10 - p. 1314

27. IN INFANT MONKEYS SEPARATED FROM THEIR MOTHERS, THE DE-
    SPAIR STAGE IS CHARACTERIZED BY THE FOLLOWING, EXCEPT:
    A. Excessive self-clasping
    B. Reduced levels of locomotion
    C. Increased huddling
    D. Increased self-mouthing
    E. Excessive vocalization   Ref. 10 - p. 1314

28. THE BLOOD LEVELS OF IMIPRAMINE AND ITS METABOLITE DES-
    METHYLIMIPRAMINE CAN BE ELEVATED BY THE ADDITION OF:
    A. Chlorpromazine
    B. Methylphenidate
    C. Methyprylon
    D. Methaqualone
    E. Diazepam   Ref. 11 - p. 1321

29. AN ADVANTAGE OF THE ABOVE COMBINED THERAPY WOULD BE:
    A. More rapid onset of a clinical response
    B. Economic advantage because of lower cost of the latter drug
    C. The possibility of suicide is reduced
    D. Recurrence of depression is unusual
    E. All of the above   Ref. 11 - p. 1326

30. AN ADVERSE REACTION TO PSYCHOTROPIC MEDICATION THAT HAS
    BEEN FOUND TO BE MORE COMMON IN WOMEN THAN IN MEN IS:
    A. Phenothiazine-induced tremors
    B. Cerebral seizures
    C. Toxic psychosis
    D. Lens opacity
    E. Agranulocytosis   Ref. 11 - p. 1341

31. ANOTHER ADVERSE REACTION TO PSYCHOTROPIC MEDICATION SEEN
    MORE COMMONLY IN WOMEN IS:
    A. Photosensitivity
    B. Urinary retention
    C. Purple skin
    D. Hypotensive reaction
    E. Paralytic ileus   Ref. 11 - p. 1343

32. TOXIC CONFUSIONAL STATES , OCCASIONALLY ASSOCIATED WITH
    VISUAL HALLUCINATIONS, CAN BE PRODUCED BY:
    A. Phenothiazines
    B. Amitrityline
    C. A combination of a phenothiazine with an antiparkinsonian drug
    D. A combination of a phenothiazine with an anticholinergic agent
    E. All of the above   Ref. 11 - p. 1342

33. THE "QUEEQUEG SYNDROME" HAS BEEN FOUND TO OCCUR:
    A. In sailors, during lengthy sea voyages
    B. Following sensory deprivation
    C. In patients discharged from mental hospitals
    D. With prolonged phenothiazine therapy
    E. In dream-deprived subjects   Ref. 12 - p. 1337

34. AN EFFECTIVE TREATMENT FOR THIS SYNDROME IS:
    A. Ascorbic acid in high doses
    B. Imipramine
    C. Therapeutic community
    D. Procyclidine
    E. Chlorpromazine   Ref. 12 - p. 1337

35. IN THE FOLLOW-UP STUDY OF WRIST SLASHERS, IMPROVEMENT:
    A. Is rare
    B. May be attributed to increased ability to verbalize feelings
    C. Is independent of psychotic guilt
    D. Is most likely if patient is not taken seriously
    E. Is independent of psychotherapeutic intervention

    Ref. 13 - p. 1347

36. SUICIDE IN WRIST SLASHERS:
    A. Is uncommon
    B. Is preventable if antidepressant medication is prescribed
    C. Is a danger if psychotic guilt is present
    D. All of the above
    E. None of the above

    Ref. 13 - p. 1348

37. THE MOST COMMON TYPICAL THEME IN BOTH EARLY MEMORIES
    AND DREAMS:
    A. Is of falling through space
    B. Is of the object endangered
    C. Relates to food and eating
    D. Concerns openly sexual matters
    E. Relates to school and work respectively

    Ref. 14 - p. 1354

38. MOST EARLY MEMORIES ARE PLACED IN TIME AS HAVING OCCURRED:
    A. At one to two years of age
    B. At three to four years of age
    C. At five to six years of age
    D. At seven to eight years of age
    E. At nine years of age and older

    Ref. 14 - p. 1356

39. THE INSTITUTION MOST FREQUENTLY REFERRED TO IN DREAMS IS:
    A. The family of origin
    B. The family of marriage
    C. The school
    D. Work
    E. The state

    Ref. 14 - p. 1355

40. DAY HOSPITAL PATIENTS GENERALLY HAVE A REHOSPITALIZATION
    RATE:
    A. That is lower than that of inpatients
    B. That is higher than that of inpatients
    C. That equals the rehospitalization rate of inpatients
    D. Which cannot be accurately measured because they are often
       unavailable for follow-up studies
    E. That varies inversely with the length of hospital stay

    Ref. 15 - p. 1377

41. DAY HOSPITALIZATION MAY BE SUPERIOR TO INPATIENT CARE:
    A. In certain cases, despite the patients being suicidal
    B. Because of higher levels of staff commitment
    C. Because it avoids the regressive features of total institutionalization
    D. For the detoxification of heroin addiction
    E. All of the above

    Ref. 15 - p. 1379

THE LENGTH OF TIME A PATIENT REMAINS IN THE DAY HOSPITAL:
A. Is always less than for inpatients, on the average
B. Is influenced by administrative policy considerations
C. May extend for years in some studies
D. Is always more than for inpatients, on the average
E. Varies directly with the readmission rate
Ref. 15 - p. 1381

PATIENTS WITH RECURRENT DEPRESSIONS WHO ARE TREATED WITH LITHIUM:
A. Rarely experience a return of depression
B. Have more frequent depressive episodes, but do not have hypomanic or manic attacks
C. Continue to experience recurrence of depression which often responds to tricyclics or MAO inhibitors
D. Should be taken off lithium if depression recurs
E. Require an increase in lithium to above maintenance levels if depression recurs
Ref. 16 - p. 1400

THE SYNDROME KNOWN AS TARDIVE DYSKINESIA:
A. Usually responds to treatment with antiparkinsonian medication
B. Tends to improve when the causative neuroleptic is removed
C. Has a direct relationship to the development of pseudoparkinsonism
D. Is associated with reduced anxiety
E. Tends to persist despite the withdrawal of drugs
Ref. 17 - p. 1410

THE SYNDROME OF MINIMAL BRAIN DYSFUNCTION IS CHARACTERIZED BY THE FOLLOWING EXCEPT:
A. Resistance to discipline
B. Emotional volatility
C. Low frustration tolerance
D. Inattentiveness and distractability
E. Decreased motor activity
Ref. 18 - p. 1411

A TREATMENT INTRODUCED BY BRADLEY IN 1937, WHICH OFTEN PRO-DUCES AMELIORATION IN CHILDREN WITH MBD SYNDROME IS:
A. Diphenylhydantoin
B. Diphenylmethanes
C. D-amphetamine
D. Dopamine
E. Methylphenidate
Ref. 18 - p. 1412

CHILDREN WITH MINIMAL BRAIN DAMAGE (MBD) HAVE BEEN FOUND TO HAVE THE FOLLOWING, EXCEPT:
A. Soft neurological signs
B. Increased EEG abnormalities
C. Disturbance on the Bender-Gestalt test
D. Difficulty in figure-ground discrimination
E. Diminished production of monoamines
Ref. 18 - p. 1414

48. THE THERAPEUTIC RESPONSE PRODUCED IN MBD CHILDREN BY AMPHETAMINES AND ANTIDEPRESSANTS SUGGESTS A FUNCTIONAL OVERPRODUCTION OF:
   A. Serotonin
   B. Dopamine
   C. Norepinephrine
   D. All of the above
   E. None of the above
   Ref. 18 - p. 1412

49. THE DESTRUCTIVE TREND IN PSYCHIATRY HIGHLIGHTED BY KUBIE IS:
   A. The failure to use phenothiazines in sufficiently high doses in the early treatment of schizophrenia
   B. Endless waiting lists in mental hygiene clinics
   C. The retreat from one to one work with patients
   D. Inadequate staffing of state mental hospitals
   E. Inadequate treatment facilities for drug addiction
   Ref. 19 - p. 98

50. A CRUCIAL FACTOR UNDERLYING THIS TREND, ACCORDING TO KUBIE IS:
   A. Inadequate training in pharmacotherapy in residency programs
   B. Lack of financial support from federal sources
   C. Preferential backing of OPD facilities by government
   D. Activation of the therapist's own unsolved problems
   E. The recent training early in medical school
   Ref. 19 - p. 103

51. ANOTHER CAUSE DESCRIBED BY KUBIE IS:
   A. Inadequate coverage by insurance companies for psychiatric illness
   B. The model of the nonclinician teacher in departments of psychiatry
   C. Too few drug treatment evaluation programs
   D. Need for greater use of methadone in treatment programs
   E. Lack of training early in medical school
   Ref. 19 - p. 100

52. EGO MECHANISMS OF DEFENSE ARE MENTAL PROCESSES THAT ARE:
   A. Habitual, unconscious, and sometimes pathological
   B. Habitual, unconscious, and always pathological
   C. Habitual, conscious or unconscious, and sometimes pathological
   D. Transient, conscious or unconscious, and pathological
   E. Transient, conscious, and pathological
   Ref. 20 - p. 107

53. THE INFERRED PURPOSE OF EGO MECHANISMS OF DEFENSE IS:
   A. Keeping affects within bearable limits
   B. Handling conflict with important people
   C. Postponing sudden increases in biological drives
   D. All of the above
   E. None of the above
   Ref. 20 - p. 107

54. DENIAL IS A DEFENSE MECHANISM WHICH IS:
    A. Less pathological than somatization
    B. More pathological than repression and less pathological than ritual
    C. More pathological than distortion and less pathological than dissociation
    D. More pathological than somatization
    E. None of the above   Ref. 20 - p. 108

55. OF THE EGO MECHANISMS OF DEFENSE, DENIAL IS ONE WHICH:
    A. Abolishes external stimuli
    B. Is used in fantasy and daydreaming
    C. Is common in psychosis
    D. May be seen in adults under very severe stress
    E. All of the above   Ref. 20 - p. 108

56. AN EXAMPLE OF A MATURE EGO MECHANISM OF DEFENSE WOULD BE:
    A. Intellectualization
    B. Acting out
    C. Sublimation
    D. Displacement
    E. Passive-aggressive behavior   Ref. 20 - p. 111

57. THE EGO MECHANISMS OF DEFENSE:
    A. Require clinical acumen to discover since they are like hidden figures camouflaged by their neutral background
    B. Are theoretical constructs
    C. Are a conceptualization which remains one of the most valuable contributions psychoanalysis has made to medicine
    D. All of the above
    E. None of the above   Ref. 20 - p. 107,115

58. AN EXAMPLE OF A NEUROTIC DEFENSE MECHANISM WOULD BE:
    A. Repression
    B. Acting out
    C. Denial
    D. Projection
    E. Anticipation   Ref. 20 - p. 111

59. NARCISSISTIC DEFENSE MECHANISMS:
    A. Are more common in children under age 5, and in adult dreams and fantasy
    B. Alter reality for the user, and appear psychotic to the observer
    C. Can be altered by phenothiazines and removal of stress
    D. Can be given up in supportive and reality-oriented psychotherapy
    E. All of the above   Ref. 20 - p. 116

60. IMMATURE DEFENSE MECHANISMS:
    A. Are common in children aged 3 to 16
    B. Occur in character and affective disorders
    C. Appear socially undesirable and may be labelled "misbehavior"
    D. All of the above
    E. None of the above   Ref. 20 - p. 116

61. ALL OF THE FOLLOWING ARE CHARACTERISTIC OF PASSIVE-AGGRES-
SIVE BEHAVIOR, EXCEPT:
   A. It is occasionally operative as a mature defense
   B. Underlying it are passivity, masochism, and turning against the self
   C. Aggression toward others is expressed indirectly
   D. It includes provocative behavior designed to attract attention
   E. Assumption of a competitive role is avoided
                                          Ref. 20 - p. 117

62. REM SLEEP CAN BE TOTALLY SUPPRESSED:
   A. In certain types of schizophrenia
   B. By high doses of chlorpromazine
   C. By the use of monoamine oxidase inhibitors
   D. When subjects are awakened frequently during the night
   E. If subjects are required to write down their dreams
                                          Ref. 21 - p. 152

63. REM SLEEP CAN BE INCREASED BY:
   A. Amphetamines
   B. Tricyclic antidepressants
   C. Monoamine oxidase inhibitors
   D. Reserpine
   E. Methylphenidate   Ref. 21 - p. 153

64. THE SUPPRESSION OF REM SLEEP MAY:
   A. Occur during the treatment of schizophrenia
   B. Help to alleviate depression
   C. Occur during pregnancy
   D. Cause convulsions
   E. Be accompanied by increased reporting of dreams
                                          Ref. 21 - p. 153

65. LINKAGE WITH THE COLOR BLINDNESS LOCUS:
   A. Tends to confirm that a disorder is linked to the Y chromosome
   B. Has been found in schizophrenia
   C. Has been found in primary affective disorders
   D. Has been found in manic-depressive disease
   E. Locates the disorder on an autosomal chromosome
                                          Ref. 22 - p. 1128

66. A PARENT WITH AN AFFECTIVE DISORDER:
   A. Is found more frequently in manic-depressive than in depressive
      patients
   B. Is found more frequently in depressive than in manic-depressive
      patients
   C. Is always found in the history of manic patients
   D. Usually has offspring with affective disorders
   E. None of the above   Ref. 22 - p. 1129

15

67. THOUGHT DISRUPTION, DEPERSONALIZATION, IMPAIRMENT OF RECENT MEMORY, INCREASED PERCEPTUAL AWARENESS, AND PARANOIA:
    A. Are drug effects reported when marijuana is used one to four times per month
    B. Occur only when marijuana is used 20 to 30 times a month
    C. Occur rarely with marijuana usage
    D. Occur only in users with a history of psychiatric disorder
    E. Occur only when multiple drugs are used
                                    Ref. 23 - p. 1138

68. HEAVY USERS OF MARIJUANA (20 TO 30 TIMES PER MONTH) TEND TO:
    A. Perform work which is below their intellectual and previous scholastic ability
    B. Have an air of self-neglect and somewhat disheveled appearance
    C. Be vague and tangential
    D. All of the above
    E. None of the above   Ref. 23 - p. 1138

69. A DRUG WHICH FREQUENTLY INDUCES VIOLENT BEHAVIOR, INCLUDING HOMICIDE, IS:
    A. Heroin
    B. Morphine
    C. Methadone
    D. Acridans
    E. Amphetamine   Ref. 24 - p. 1170

70. CHARACTERISTIC OF THE POPULATION ABUSING METHEDRINE IS(ARE):
    A. High incidence of withdrawal seizures
    B. Possession of knives, pistols, and rifles
    C. Development of drug tolerance is unusual
    D. Feelings of inferiority
    E. Avoidance of intravenous use   Ref. 24 - p. 1174

71. THE COMBINATION OF AMPHETAMINES WITH ALCOHOL AND SEDATIVES:
    A. Tends to be avoided by those in the drug sub-culture
    B. Leads to memory loss for the assaultive behavior
    C. Leads to decreased amounts of amphetamine being used
    D. Causes the user to sleep for prolonged periods
    E. May improve impulse control   Ref. 24 - p. 1173

72. A UNIVERSAL PHENOMENON IN PATIENTS FOLLOWING RENAL TRANSPLANTATION IS:
    A. Denial
    B. Projection
    C. Internalization
    D. Undoing
    E. Intellectualization   Ref. 25 - p. 1188

73. THE INCIDENCE OF SUICIDAL BEHAVIOR IN CHRONIC HEMODIALYSIS PATIENTS IS:
    A. Higher in home dialysis compared to hospital dialysis patients
    B. Double that of the general population
    C. Higher in women than in men
    D. All of the above
    E. None of the above   Ref. 26 - p. 1200

74. COMPETENCY TO STAND TRIAL:
    A. Is a decision based on the M'Naghten Rules
    B. Can be determined by the Durham ruling
    C. Is decided by the Briggs Law
    D. Must be decided by a court-appointed psychiatrist
    E. Is ultimately a judicial judgment   Ref. 27 - p. 1226

75. CRITERIA OF COMPETENCY TO STAND TRIAL INCLUDE:
    A. Cooperation and participation in own defense
    B. Current absence of mental illness
    C. Requirement for hospitalization
    D. All of the above
    E. None of the above   Ref. 27 - p. 1229

76. A SIGN FOUND IN PREGNANCY BUT NOT IN PSEUDOCYESIS IS:
    A. Amenorrhea
    B. Effacement of the umbilicus
    C. Abdominal enlargement
    D. Breast changes
    E. Enlargement of the uterus   Ref. 28 - p. 221

77. A DEFINITIVE DIAGNOSIS OF PSEUDOCYESIS CAN BE MADE BY:
    A. Reversal of abdominal enlargement under anesthesia
    B. Levels of urinary gonadotropin
    C. Friedman pregnancy test
    D. Evaluation of size of uterus
    E. All of the above   Ref. 28 - p. 221

78. A COMPARISON OF THE DEPRESSIVE STATE IN UNIPOLAR VERSUS
    BIPOLAR AFFECTIVE ILLNESS REVEALS THAT:
    A. The unipolar patient is more active when depressed
    B. The bipolar patient is more active when depressed
    C. The unipolar patient shows retardation and seclusive behavior
    D. Pacing is characteristic of bipolar patients
    E. Overt expression of anger is higher in bipolar patients
       Ref. 29 - p. 219

79. UNIPOLAR AFFECTIVE ILLNESS PATIENTS HAVE MORE FREQUENTLY
    THAN BIPOLAR PATIENTS:
    A. An earlier age of onset of depressive episode
    B. Positive response to lithium
    C. Higher incidence of celibacy (males) and divorce
    D. Higher incidence of parental loss prior to age 13
    E. Presence of precipitating factors for recurrences following the first
       episode of depression   Ref. 29 - p. 218

80. IN HIS WORK WITH SCHIZOPHRENICS, LAING HAS DEMONSTRATED
    THAT:
    A. Vigorous treatment with phenothiazines is necessary for social recovery
    B. Cultural factors shape the thought disorder
    C. The patient attempts to describe his actual social situation in his
       incoherent speech
    D. Social class is a factor in the development of mental illness
    E. Mental illness is more frequent in London than in rural parts of
       England   Ref. 30 - p. 207

81. STUDIES WHICH FOCUS ON SOCIAL FACTORS IN SCHIZOPHRENIA
ENCOMPASS:
A. Epidemiological studies
B. Family interactional studies
C. Cross-cultural studies
D. All of the above
E. None of the above   Ref. 30 - p. 207

82. FARIS AND DUNHAM'S WORK ON MENTAL DISORDERS IN URBAN AREAS
DEMONSTRATED:
A. That heroin addiction is more prevalent in ghetto areas
B. An increase of addiction in suburbs in the last 20 years
C. A relationship between economic and cultural impoverishment and
rates of specific mental diseases
D. That the rate of schizophrenia is lower in cities
E. Familial skew   Ref. 30 - p. 208

83. THE WORK OF LIDZ AND HIS GROUP AT YALE:
A. Attempts a conceptualization of the kind of family setting that leads to
development of schizophrenia in the child
B. Led to the development of the double-bind theory
C. Is based on the view of schizophrenia as a hereditary disease
D. Has found that biochemical disorders exist in process schizophrenia
E. Considers that one family type leads to schizophrenia
Ref. 30 - p. 210

84. CULTURAL FACTORS WHICH POSSIBLY LEAD TO PRODUCING MENTAL
ILLNESS INCLUDE:
A. Child-rearing practices
B. Processes of cultural change
C. Cultural patterns of breeding
D. Cultural patterns of poor physical hygiene
E. All of the above   Ref. 30 - p. 212

85. A CENTRAL CONCEPT IN THE THEORY OF GEORGE HERBERT MEAD IS:
A. The influence of culture on sexual attitudes
B. The evolving of the self (the "I" and the "me")
C. Pseudomutuality
D. Double-bind
E. Familial skew   Ref. 30 - p. 210

86. THE STIRLING COUNTY STUDY CONFIRMED:
A. That half-way houses can be an alternative to state hospital custodial
care
B. The relationship between high prevalence of mental disorder and the
condition known as sociocultural disintegration
C. That mental disorder and social class are inversely related
D. The effectiveness of walk-in clinics
E. The superiority of day-hospital to full-time inpatient care
Ref. 31 - p. 244

87. WHITE DEFINES "COMPETENCE" AS:
    A. The ability to do one's work with satisfaction and effectiveness
    B. The capacity to fulfill one's role in the family setting
    C. The ability of therapist to diagnose and treat his patients competently
    D. The capacity of the organism to interact effectively with its environment
    E. The capacity to empathize   Ref. 31 - p. 253

88. AGRANULOCYTOSIS IS:
    A. Rarely fatal
    B. Preventable if routine monthly WBC examination is performed
    C. Associated with fever and ulceration of mucous membranes of oropharynx
    D. Not associated with benzodiazepines
    E. Not associated with tricyclics   Ref. 32 - p. 265

89. JANUSIAN THINKING REFERS TO:
    A. The capacity to utilize opposite ideas simultaneously
    B. The schizophrenic thought disorder
    C. Predicative identification
    D. Thought processes brought about by the double-bind
    E. Ambivalence   Ref. 33 - p. 195

90. JANUSIAN THINKING IS PRESENT IN:
    A. Schizophrenogenic parents
    B. Oneirophrenic states
    C. Organic mental syndromes
    D. LSD intoxication
    E. The act of creation   Ref. 33 - p. 203

91. FREQUENT IN THE HISTORY OF MEN WITH TRANSVESTISM IS AN
    EPISODE OF:
    A. Being dressed in female clothing in childhood by a man
    B. Sexual seduction by an older female relative
    C. Being dressed in female clothing in childhood by a woman
    D. Homosexual seduction before the age of 12
    E. Incest   Ref. 34 - p. 232

92. TRANSVESTISM (FETISHISTIC CROSS-DRESSING):
    A. Occurs more often in woman
    B. Is found in men who are usually overtly homosexual
    C. Is rare in married men
    D. Occurs in men who are generally effeminate in other behavior
    E. Produces genital excitation in those with this symptom
              Ref. 34 - p. 231

93. TRANSSEXUALISM IN MALES:
    A. Leads to an incapacity for sexual relations with women
    B. Leads to a sexual preference for homosexual men
    C. Is not associated with a wish for surgical sexual transformation
    D. Is identical with transvestism
    E. Is characterized by sexual excitement induced by garments
              Ref. 34 - p. 232

94. EFFEMINATE HOMOSEXUAL MEN WHO CROSS-DRESS:
    A. Often request surgical sexual transformation
    B. Do not experience sexual excitement induced by the clothes
    C. Do not prefer men as sexual objects
    D. All of the above
    E. None of the above   Ref. 34 - p. 233

95. INCREASED INCIDENCE OF CHROMOSOMAL ABERRATIONS HAS BEEN
    REPORTED:
    A. In psychiatric patients treated with phenothiazines
    B. In subjects who have taken LSD
    C. In heroin addicts
    D. All of the above
    E. None of the above   Ref. 35 - p. 270

96. LIFTON'S CONCEPT OF PROTEAN MAN REFERS TO:
    A. A personality style characterized by constant shifts in identification
    B. Pathological reactions in atomic bomb survivors
    C. Delayed reactions in concentration camp victims
    D. Personality disturbances following use of marijuana
    E. Sequelae of permissive upbringing   Ref. 36 - p. 298

97. URINARY EXCRETION OF CYCLIC AMP IS ELEVATED IN:
    A. Mania
    B. Depression
    C. Patients whose mania improved on lithium
    D. Patients whose mania improved on chlorpromazine
    E. Schizophrenia   Ref. 37 - p. 327

98. THE PROGNOSIS IN MANIC-DEPRESSIVE ILLNESS IS MORE FAVORABLE:
    A. In those patients with depressive attacks only
    B. In those patients with manic attacks only
    C. In patients with manic and depressive attacks
    D. In women than in men   Ref. 38 - p. 334

99. THE MEAN DURATION OF A MANIC-DEPRESSIVE ATTACK IS:
    A. Two months
    B. Four months
    C. Eight months
    D. One year
    E. Two years   Ref. 38 - p. 336

100. THE MEAN DURATION OF SYMPTOM-FREE INTERVALS IN MANIC-
     DEPRESSIVE ILLNESS IS:
     A. One year
     B. Two years
     C. Three years
     D. Six years
     E. Twelve years   Ref. 38 - p. 336

101. SHORT SLEEPERS AND LONG SLEEPERS SPEND AN IDENTICAL AMOUNT
     OF TIME:
     A. In REM sleep
     B. In Stage 1
     C. In Stage 2
     D. In Stage 3
     E. In Stage 3 and 4   Ref. 39 - p. 1004

102. SHORT SLEEPERS AND LONG SLEEPERS SPEND A SIMILAR PERCENT-
AGE OF THEIR TIME IN BED IN:
A. REM sleep
B. Stage 1
C. Stage 2
D. Stage 3
E. Stage 3 and 4   Ref. 39 - p. 1005

103. THE SUGGESTION THAT SLOW WAVE SLEEP (STAGE 3 AND 4) HAS AN
ANABOLIC OR PHYSICALLY RESTORATIVE FUNCTION IS BASED ON:
A. Peaks of human growth hormone occurring during slow wave sleep
B. It being relatively constant for all subjects
C. Its amount being altered by exercise
D. All of the above
E. None of the above   Ref. 39 - p. 1007

104. REM SLEEP (D STATE) TIME TENDS TO BE LOW IN:
A. Women with premenstrual tension
B. Mania
C. Times of psychic disequilibrium with changing defense patterns
D. Long sleepers
E. All of the above   Ref. 39 - p. 1007

105. SHORT SLEEPERS TEND TO BE:
A. Efficient and hardworking
B. Somewhat depressed
C. Anxious
D. Withdrawn
E. Relatively high in incidence of mental illness
                                    Ref. 39 - p. 1001

106. LONG SLEEPERS TEND TO BE:
A. Hypomanic
B. Manic
C. Anxious, depressed and withdrawn
D. Good sleepers as regards efficiency of sleep
E. More intelligent than short sleepers   Ref. 39 - p. 1001

107. THE NEED FOR D SLEEP (REM SLEEP):
A. Has not been demonstrated conclusively
B. Varies from individual to individual
C. Does not appear to be related to personality or psychological state
D. Is high in manic states
E. Is greater than the need for slow wave sleep
                                    Ref. 39 - p. 1007

108. THE EFFECT OF IMIPRAMINE ON NOREPINEPHRINE TURNOVER IN
BRAIN:
A. Turnover is slowed after chronic administration of imipramine
B. Turnover is increased after single dose of imipramine
C. Thyroid hormone decelerates the norepinephrine turnover
D. May explain delay in antidepressant effect with imipramine
E. There is no effect   Ref. 40 - p. 1032

109. A MEANS OF ACCELERATING AND ENHANCING THE ANTIDEPRESSANT
EFFECT OF IMIPRAMINE IS:
A. Concomitant use of insulin
B. Combination with chlorpromazine
C. Perphenazine
D. Thyroid hormone
E. Lithium   Ref. 40 - p. 1038

110. LENTICULAR AND CORNEAL OPACITIES SECONDARY TO CHLOR-
PROMAZINE:
A. Generally do not cause visual impairment
B. Are not related to total intake of the drug
C. Are often associated with retinal involvement
D. Are usually reversible
E. Are rare   Ref. 41 - p. 1045

111. CONCERNING THE RELATIONSHIP BETWEEN EYE OPACITIES AND
NEUROLEPTICS OTHER THAN CHLORPROMAZINE:
A. Levomepromazine is a neuroleptic that also causes such changes
B. Most other neuroleptics have not been reported to cause such changes
C. Patients receive smaller doses of other neuroleptics than the doses
of chlorpromazine, and there is, therefore, less likelihood of opacity
formation
D. All of the above
E. None of the above   Ref. 41 - p. 1045

112. FOR THE MANAGEMENT OF PATIENTS RECEIVING HIGH DOSES OF
CHLORPROMAZINE:
A. It would be important to be aware that exposure to UV light may lead
to development of epithelial keratopathy (opacity of corneal surface)
B. Penlight may be used to detect opacities of the lens
C. It is recommended that they be screened for eye opacities after
accumulating 300 to 400 grams of phenothiazine
D. All of the above
E. None of the above   Ref. 41 - p. 1048

113. AN EFFECTIVE TREATMENT FOR THE DELIRIUM OFTEN CAUSED BY
ANTICHOLINERGICS IS:
A. Procyclidine and chlorpromazine
B. Physostigmine
C. Atropine
D. Scopolamine
E. Hyoscyamine   Ref. 42 - p. 1050

114. DELIRIUM SECONDARY TO ANTICHOLINERGIC DRUGS MAY FOLLOW:
A. Preoperative medication
B. Antiparkinsonian drugs
C. Non-prescription drugs used for sleeping (e.g., Sleep-Eze and Sominex)
D. Eye drops
E. All of the above   Ref. 42 - p. 1050

22

115. PYRIDOXINE IS CAPABLE OF REVERSING THE CHOREIFORM DYSKINESIA:
   A. Associated with prolonged use of phenothiazines (tardive dyskinesia)
   B. Huntington's chorea manifest
   C. Secondary to L-dopa therapy
   D. All of the above
   E. None of the above   Ref. 43 - p. 1091

116. KUBIE POINTS OUT THAT THE USE OF HUMOR IN PSYCHOTHERAPY IS:
   A. Usually contraindicated
   B. Often effective
   C. Helpful in the bantering form used by Sullivan
   D. A therapeutic means of coping with countertransferential anger
   E. Indicated in the psychotherapy of depression
                                  Ref. 44 - p. 861

117. ZETZEL HAS RECOMMENDED THAT THE BORDERLINE PATIENT BE TREATED WITH:
   A. Tricyclic antidepressant drugs
   B. Phenothiazines in the moderate to high dose range
   C. Intensive psychotherapy several times per week
   D. Regular but limited contact very seldom more than once a week
   E. The resources of community psychiatry
                                  Ref. 45 - p. 870

118. DIRECT TESTING OF NOREPINEPHRINE, SEROTONIN, AND DOPAMINE IN MAN FOR CONFIRMATION OF THE BIOGENIC AMINE THEORY OF MANIA AND DEPRESSION:
   A. Has demonstrated the validity of the theory
   B. Has been performed but the results contradict the theory
   C. Is not possible because of their toxicity
   D. Cannot be done because they do not pass the blood-brain barrier
   E. Leads to equivocal results   Ref. 46 - p. 872

119. A DRUG WHICH PASSES THE BLOOD-BRAIN BARRIER AND INHIBITS SYNTHESIS OF NOREPINEPHRINE OR SEROTONIN:
   A. Would be expected to decrease manic symptoms
   B. Would likely cause improvement in depression
   C. Exists, which inhibits serotonin, but none inhibits epinephrine synthesis
   D. Does not exist
   E. Leads to rise in urinary VMA   Ref. 46 - p. 873

120. A DRUG WHICH INCREASES LEVELS OF NOREPINEPHRINE, SEROTONIN, AND DOPAMINE IS:
   A. Alpha-methyl-para-tyrosine
   B. Parachlorophenylalanine
   C. Imipramine
   D. Chlorpromazine
   E. Reserpine   Ref. 46 - p. 872

121. A SIGNIFICANT FINDING IN THE HISTORY OF HOMICIDAL ADOLESCENTS IS:
   A. Divorce or separation of parents
   B. Ghetto environment
   C. Parental brutality
   D. Death of a parent before the patient is 12 years old
   E. Parental rejection   Ref. 47 - p. 1500

122. "FLOODING" (IMPLOSIVE THERAPY) IS A TREATMENT MODALITY:
    A. Designed for the treatment of character disorders
    B. Which involves presentation of a hierarchy of fear situations
    C. Forcing the patient to remain in a prolonged state of sleep
    D. Forcing abstinence from all gratification
    E. Preventing avoidance response in presence of full strength fear
       stimuli   Ref. 48 - p. 1509

123. AUTOKINESIS REFERS TO:
    A. The basis for behavior disorder in children
    B. Apparent motion of a pinpoint of light in a dark room
    C. Extinction of conditioned fear
    D. A hypnagogic phenomenon
    E. Delayed toxic effect of phenothiazines
                                         Ref. 49 - p. 1515

124. PERSONS WHO EXPERIENCE VERY LITTLE OR NO AUTOKINESIS:
    A. Are more vulnerable to external stimuli
    B. Are found in the manic-depressive diagnostic category
    C. Are more likely to require hospitalization when psychiatrically ill
    D. All of the above
    E. None of the above   Ref. 49 - p. 1518

125. IN PERSONS WITH EARLY TOTAL DEAFNESS IT IS RARE TO ENCOUNTER:
    A. Psychotic depressions with psychomotor retardation
    B. Paranoid reactions
    C. Impulsive, aggressive behavior
    D. Auditory hallucinations in those with schizophrenia
    E. Egocentricity   Ref. 50 - p. 1523

126. BASED ON FINDINGS IN PERSONS WITH EARLY TOTAL DEAFNESS, IT
    IS REASONABLE TO HYPOTHESIZE THAT AUDITION IS NECESSARY
    FOR:
    A. Formation of paranoid ideation
    B. Development of obsessional character
    C. Development of hysterical character
    D. Formation of auditory hallucinations
    E. Development of schizophrenia   Ref. 50 - p. 1525

127. THE MOST COMMON INITIAL REACTION OF RECENTLY BLIND ADULTS
    IS:
    A. Paranoid ideation
    B. Depression
    C. Shame
    D. Guilt
    E. Anger   Ref. 51 - p. 1534

128. ADULTS WHO HAVE RECENTLY BECOME BLIND:
    A. Rarely are able to recall their dreams
    B. Generally go through an initial period during which they experience
       visual hallucinations
    C. May experience complete denial of blindness(anosognosia)
    D. All of the above
    E. None of the above   Ref. 51 - pp. 1534, 1536

129. A RARE CONDITION WHICH HAS A RELATIVELY HIGH INCIDENCE IN
CONGENITALLY BLIND CHILDREN IS:
A. Infantile neurosis
B. Infantile autism
C. Symbiotic psychosis
D. Lesch-Nyhan syndrome
E. Freeman-Sheldon (Whistling Face) syndrome
Ref. 52 - p. 1539

130. ALTHOUGH INFANTS WHO ARE BLIND DO NOT REACH OUT FOR SOUND-
MAKING OBJECTS UNTIL THEY ARE ABOUT TEN MONTHS OLD:
A. They can be shown to discriminate their mothers' voices at ten weeks
B. This is not a developmental lag based on CNS pathology
C. Sighted infants who do not make visual contact with a sound source
at once lose interest in it and do not reach out either
D. All infants appear to require to be nine or ten months before using
sound for cognitive purposes
E. All of the above
Ref. 52 - p. 1541

131. MANIC-DEPRESSIVE PATIENTS WHO HAVE BEEN TREATED WITH
LITHIUM:
A. Often do well when lithium is withdrawn following some months of
treatment
B. Should be withdrawn from lithium following abatement of the manic
attack since lithium is not approved for prophylaxis by the FDA
C. Should remain on the drug indefinitely if there is no untoward toxicity
and clinical benefit appears to continue
D. May no longer require frequent monitoring of plasma lithium levels
once they have been stabilized
E. Do not require regular outpatient follow-up
Ref. 53 - p. 1558

132. LITHIUM TREATMENT IS ASSOCIATED WITH:
A. Leukocytosis
B. Leukopenia
C. Agranulocytosis
D. Jaundice
E. Parkinsonian tremor
Ref. 54 - p. 1559

133. CHILDREN WHO ARE NOT FIRST-BORN:
A. Tend to have greater father-son contact than do first-borns
B. Are more frequently found in the ranks of jet-pilots
C. Score higher in tests of intelligence
D. All of the above
E. None of the above
Ref. 55 - p. 735

134. UNILATERAL ECT IS LIKELY TO RESULT IN REDUCED:
A. Number of treatment sessions
B. Anesthetic exposure time
C. Number of treatment failures
D. Memory dysfunction during the immediate treatment period
E. Relapse rate
Ref. 56 - p. 744

135. THE EPIDEMIOLOGICAL CHARACTERISTICS OF THE SERIOUS-ATTEMPT
     GROUP OF THOSE WHO ATTEMPT SUICIDE REVEAL THAT:
     A. There are relatively few with manic-depressive depression
     B. Most are under 30
     C. Use of barbiturates is uncommon
     D. Insomnia is significant
     E. Depression is not significant   Ref. 57 - p. 768

136. THE INCREASE IN ACTIVITY OF SERUM CREATINE PHOSPHOKINASE
     (CPK) TYPE III IN ACUTELY PSYCHOTIC PATIENTS SUGGESTS:
     A. Presence of a myopathy
     B. CNS disorder
     C. Cardiac disturbance
     D. Liver disease
     E. Decreased physical exercise   Ref. 58 - p. 488

137. THE ALKALINE-PHOSPHATASE-POSITIVE FIBER IS USEFUL IN
     IDENTIFYING:
     A. Neuropathies
     B. Thyroid abnormality
     C. Alzheimer's syndrome
     D. Wernicke's syndrome
     E. Myopathy   Ref. 59 - p. 493

138. THE VERBAL HOSTILITY SCORE IN THE BUSS-DURKEE INVENTORY:
     A. Is increased during depression
     B. Is increased following improvement from depression
     C. Is decreased following improvement from depression
     D. Does not change after depression is ameliorated
     E. Measures introjected aggression   Ref. 60 - p. 534

139. AGORAPHOBIA:
     A. Is more common in women
     B. Rarely occurs in young adults
     C. Can often be cured by high motivation
     D. Usually clears within a year
     E. Rarely is associated with depression
                                              Ref. 61 - p. 552

140. NEUROLOGICAL HYPERSENSITIVITY TO PSYCHOTROPIC DRUGS,
     PARTICULARLY THOSE WITH A PIPERAZINYL SIDE CHAIN OCCURS:
     A. In depression
     B. Following ECT
     C. With the associated use of amitriptyline
     D. Following lobotomy
     E. In mania   Ref. 62 - p. 596

141. THE "PINK SPOT" OR URINARY 3, 4-DIMETHOXYPHENYLETHYLAMINE
     (DMPEA) IS FOUND IN THE PRESENCE OF:
     A. Schizophrenia
     B. Acute phase of a psychosis
     C. Marijuana
     D. Heroin
     E. Tea   Ref. 63 - p. 615

142. CHILDREN WITH SCHOLASTIC-BEHAVIORAL PROBLEMS BUT NO CLASSI-
CAL EVIDENCE OF NEUROLOGICAL DISEASE DIFFER FROM CONTROLS
IN:
   A. Scores on perceptual-motor tasks
   B. Slow wave activity in their EEGs
   C. Incidence of neurological soft signs
   D. Incidence of abnormal transient discharges in sleep EEGs
   E. All of the above   Ref. 64 - p. 644

143. A NEUROLOGICAL SIGN WHICH IS NOT A "SOFT" SIGN IS:
   A. Lateral nystagmoid jerks
   B. Pupil which responds to accommodation but not to light
   C. Dysdiadochokinesis
   D. Unilateral winking defect
   E. Swaying in Romberg position   Ref. 64 - p. 636

144. HYPERACTIVE CHILDREN WITH SCHOLASTIC-BEHAVIORAL PROBLEMS
DIFFER FROM THOSE WHO ARE NONHYPERACTIVE IN HAVING:
   A. Excess number of soft neurological signs
   B. Slow activity in the EEG
   C. Perceptual-motor deficits
   D. All of the above
   E. None of the above   Ref. 64 - p. 644

145. THE LESCH-NYHAN SYNDROME INCLUDES ALL OF THE FOLLOWING
EXCEPT:
   A. Decreased concentration of uric acid in the blood
   B. Bizarre self-mutilation
   C. Aggressive behavior
   D. Spastic cerebral palsy and choreo-athetosis
   E. Developmental retardation   Ref. 65 - p. 672

146. GENETICALLY, THE LESCH-NYHAN SYNDROME IS CHARACTERIZED BY
ALL OF THE FOLLOWING, EXCEPT:
   A. It is transmitted as an X-linked recessive character trait
   B. It is a disease of the female
   C. It is a disease of the male
   D. The defect is a deficiency of HG-PRTase (hypoxanthine-guanine
      phosphoribosyl-transferase)
   E. Parents do not have the syndrome   Ref. 65 - p. 672

147. PATIENTS WITH LESCH-NYHAN SYNDROME:
   A. Have poorly coordinated eye movements
   B. Tend to relate well to those who make the effort to relate to them
   C. Exhibit surprising manual dexterity
   D. Are able to run with unusual speed
   E. Can control self-mutilation with ease if encouraged
                                            Ref. 65 - p. 672

148. THE EFFECT OF HALLUCINOGENIC DRUGS ON AUTOMOBILE DRIVING IS:
   A. Minimal if the drug is not taken while driving
   B. Present even if the person is not high because of the "flashback" pheno-
      menon or recurrences
   C. A tendency to be more careful when driving because of heightened sen-
      sitivity to stimuli
   D. Depth perception is affected but judgment is not affected
   E. Not a cause for concern for the other driver
                                            Ref. 66 - p. 685

149. THE OCULAR LESIONS PRODUCED BY HIGH DOSES OF CHLORPROMA-
      ZINE WHICH ARE REVERSIBLE ARE THOSE OF THE:
      A. Anterior cornea
      B. Posterior cornea
      C. Lens
      D. Retina
      E. Optic nerve   Ref. 67 - p. 468

150. THE CONCORDANCE RATE FOR SCHIZOPHRENIA IN MONOZYGOTIC
      TWINS IN RECENT SCANDINAVIAN AND NATIONAL ACADEMY OF
      SCIENCES-NATIONAL RESEARCH COUNCIL STUDIES:
      A. Has confirmed the findings of Kallman's study (85% concordance)
      B. Cannot be compared with Kallman's findings because of population
          differences
      C. Is much lower than the concordance rate found by Kallman
      D. Is no different from that of dizygotic twins
      E. Is higher than that found by Kallman   Ref. 68 - p. 472

151. THE CONCORDANCE RATE OF MONOZYGOTIC TWINS FOR SCHIZO-
      PHRENIA IN THE NATIONAL ACADEMY OF SCIENCES-NATIONAL
      RESEARCH COUNCIL TWIN PANEL WAS:
      A. 5%
      B. 15%
      C. 50%
      D. 85%
      E. 95%   Ref. 68 - p. 476

152. THE CONCORDANCE RATE OF MONOZYGOTIC COMPARED TO DIZYGOT-
      IC TWINS FOR SCHIZOPHRENIA IN THE NAS-NRC STUDY WAS:
      A. Five times higher
      B. Three times higher
      C. Twice as high
      D. The same
      E. Lower   Ref. 68 - p. 476

153. IN THE NAS-NRC TWIN PANEL STUDY, MONOZYGOTIC TWINS HAVE:
      A. An incidence of schizophrenia which is not significantly different
          from that in dizygotic twins
      B. A greater chance of becoming schizophrenic than a dizygotic twin
      C. A psychiatric morbidity similar to dizygotic twins
      D. Concordance rate similar to that of dizygotic twins for schizophrenia
      E. All of the above   Ref. 68 - p. 476

154. DRUG USE AMONG UNITED STATES SOLDIERS IN VIET NAM:
      A. Involves over 25% of men
      B. Is in inverse ratio to educational background
      C. Involves the use of marijuana as the drug of choice
      D. All of the above
      E. None of the above   Ref. 69 - p. 422

155. UNILATERAL ECT APPLIED TO THE DOMINANT HEMISPHERE SHOULD
BE AVOIDED:
   A. Because it is ineffective in relieving depression
   B. Because of the high amount of anesthetic required
   C. When succinylcholine is used
   D. Since the effects are more short-lived than treatment applied to
      the nondominant hemisphere
   E. Because of its effect on memory   Ref. 70 - p. 435

156. THE FINDINGS OF THE NATIONAL ACADEMY OF SCIENCES-NATIONAL
RESEARCH COUNCIL TWIN STUDY:
   A. Support the hypothesis that greater diffusion of ego boundaries and
      confusion of identity in twins is significant for development of
      schizophrenia
   B. Revealed a higher incidence of schizophrenia in monozygotic compared
      to dizygotic twins
   C. Showed schizophrenia to be having a higher incidence in twins than
      in the general population
   D. All of the above
   E. None of the above   Ref. 71 - p. 441

157. AN ASPECT OF TWINSHIP THAT COULD RESULT IN GREATER PROTEC-
TION AGAINST SCHIZOPHRENIA IS:
   A. Diffusion of ego boundaries
   B. Confusion of identity
   C. Neutralization of the "double bind"
   D. All of the above
   E. None of the above   Ref. 71 - p. 440

158. ALTERED CATECHOLAMINE EXCRETION OCCURS IN:
   A. Oral contraceptive therapy
   B. Third trimester of pregnancy
   C. Depression
   D. All of the above
   E. None of the above   Ref. 72 - p. 448

159. POOR RESPONSE TO LITHIUM TENDS TO BE CORRELATED WITH:
   A. Pre-lithium use of phenothiazines
   B. Unipolar manic disorder
   C. Length of time patient has experienced manic-depressive disorder
   D. Adverse reaction to environmental stress
   E. Presence of bipolar disorder   Ref. 73 - p. 478

160 THE MOST COMMON CARDIAC ARRHYTHMIA ASSOCIATED WITH EST IS:
   A. Premature ventricular contractions
   B. Atrial fibrillation
   C. Ventricular fibrillation
   D. Bradycardia
   E. Heart block   Ref. 74 - p. 530

161. AN EFFECTIVE TREATMENT FOR THE ABOVE ARRHYTHMIA IS:
   A. Atropine
   B. Digitalis
   C. Thiazides
   D. Succinylcholine
   E. Lidocaine   Ref. 74 - p. 530

29

162. FOLLOW-UP STUDY OF HYPERACTIVE CHILDREN REVEALS:
A. Hyperactivity generally continues through adolescence as chief complaint
B. Disorders of attention and concentration remain
C. School performance reaches a good achievement level
D. No significant psychopathology
E. Rare antisocial behavior   Ref. 75 - p. 414

163. IN IDENTICAL TWINS DISCORDANT FOR SCHIZOPHRENIA THE STRONGEST INTRA-PAIR ASSOCIATION IS BETWEEN CLINICALLY DIAGNOSED SCHIZOPHRENIA AND:
A. Maternal deprivation
B. Occurrence of neurological signs
C. Birth order
D. Parental rejection
E. Socioeconomic status   Ref. 76 - p. 427

164. THESE FINDINGS TEND TO SUGGEST:
A. That schizophrenia is a hereditary disease
B. The influence of a schizophrenogenic mother is critical
C. The "double bind" hypothesis has validity
D. Social conditions play a role in the development of schizophrenia
E. None of the above   Ref. 76 - p. 422

165. THESE FINDINGS DEMONSTRATE THE IMPORTANCE FOR THE STUDY OF SCHIZOPHRENIA OF:
A. Genetic counseling
B. Psychosocial research
C. Neurological examination
D. Family therapy
E. Intensive psychotherapeutic intervention in early childhood
          Ref. 76 - p. 422

166. ADULT SCHIZOPHRENICS WITH RELATIVELY LOW IQ SCORES:
A. Respond more poorly to insulin coma treatment
B. Tend to have an unfavorable posthospital adjustment
C. More commonly have unimproved hospital discharge ratings
D. All of the above
E. None of the above   Ref. 77 - p. 431

167. SCHIZOPHRENICS WITH LOW CHILDHOOD IQ SCORES:
A. Show an earlier age of onset
B. Have a shorter period of institutionalization compared to those with average IQ scores
C. Tend to have paranoid symptoms predominantly
D. All of the above
E. None of the above   Ref. 77 - p. 435

168. "A" AND "B" THERAPISTS HAVE BEEN SO RATED ACCORDING TO:
A. Their social class of origin
B. Use of psychotherapy versus physical methods of treatment
C. Improvement rate of their schizophrenic patients
D. Medical and non-medical training
E. Experience   Ref. 78 - p. 465

169. FIELD-DEPENDENT PATIENTS:
   A. Tend to manifest more feelings of guilt than shame
   B. Tend to have a greater number of verbal exchanges in therapy
   C. Are rare
   D. Cannot be distinguished by the rod and frame test
   E. Do not improve   Ref. 78 - p. 465

170. THE ROD AND FRAME TEST:
   A. Consistently predicts therapeutic success
   B. Measures field-dependence and field-independence
   C. Is diagnostic of psychosis
   D. Measures motivation for treatment
   E. Has been discredited   Ref. 78 - p. 466

171. SATELLITE CLINICS:
   A. Are often hospital-based and open in the evening for those who work
   B. Are neighborhood-based and respond to the needs of the disadvantaged
      urban community
   C. Have been designed for isolated rural populations
   D. Offer services unavailable in medical centers
   E. Tend to have low patient accessiblity
                                           Ref. 79 - p. 474

172. CORTISOL PRODUCTION IS HIGHEST IN DEPRESSED PATIENTS WHO
   ARE:
   A. Undergoing acute psychotic decompensation
   B. Anxious
   C. Apathetic
   D. Dejected
   E. Sad   Ref. 80 - p. 296

173. MEASUREMENT OF SUSTAINED ADRENOCORTICAL FUNCTION IS MOST
   ACCURATELY OBTAINED BY:
   A. Cortisol tagged with carbon 14 measured in the urine
   B. Daily measures of plasma cortisol
   C. 24-hour urinary excretion of 17-OHCS
   D. Sum of THE, THF, and ATHF
   E. Porter Silber reaction   Ref. 80 - p. 290

174. HIGH ELEVATIONS OF CORTICOSTEROIDS WOULD BE EXPECTED IN:
   A. Acute schizophrenic patients in psychotic turmoil
   B. Heroin addicts who are "nodding"
   C. Apathetic depressions
   D. Obesity
   E. Hysterical paralysis   Ref. 80 - p. 297

175. AN INCREASED SENSITIVITY TO ENDOGENOUS AND EXOGENOUS
   INSULIN IS RELATED TO:
   A. Depression
   B. Mania
   C. Improvement following lithium therapy
   D. Serum lithium levels
   E. Mood changes   Ref. 81 - p. 318

176. FORGETTING WHAT ONE IS GOING TO SAY NEXT AND TANGENTIALITY
OF SPEECH BECAUSE THE LINE OF THOUGHT IS LOST IS FOUND:
   A. In alcohol intoxication
   B. With LSD
   C. Following lithium therapy
   D. With marijuana
   E. With amphetamines   Ref. 82 - p. 323

177. THE FOLLOWING ARE EGO FUNCTIONS, EXCEPT:
   A. Reality testing
   B. Judgment
   C. Anxiety
   D. Sense of reality
   E. Object relations   Ref. 83 - p. 326

178. WHICH OF THE FOLLOWING IS NOT AN EGO FUNCTION?:
   A. Regulation and control of drives
   B. Dependency
   C. Thought processes
   D. Adaptive regression in the service of the ego
   E. Synthetic function   Ref. 83 - p. 326

179. EGO FUNCTIONS TEND TO BE MOST DISTURBED IN:
   A. Childhood
   B. Adolescence
   C. Schizophrenia
   D. Neurosis
   E. Character disorder   Ref. 83 - p. 335

180. HYSTERICAL PSYCHOSIS:
   A. Has an acute onset
   B. Has no schizophrenic thought disorder present
   C. Appears to be associated with anxiety related to death and actual
      object loss
   D. Is associated with object relations of a child-like quality
   E. All of the above   Ref. 84 - p. 281

181. THE AUDITORY HALLUCINATIONS IN ACUTE ALCOHOLIC PSYCHOSES:
   A. Are similar to those in schizophrenia
   B. Are more poorly localized in space than those in schizophrenia
   C. Have a cognitive taint
   D. Are better localized than those in schizophrenia
   E. Are less attention-demanding   Ref. 85 - p. 301

182. HALLUCINATIONS ARE INVARIABLY EXPERIENCED AS "TALKING TO"
THE SUBJECT IN:
   A. Schizophrenia
   B. Alcoholic hallucinosis
   C. Hysterical psychosis
   D. Marijuana intoxication
   E. Cocaine intoxication   Ref. 85 - p. 301

183. BLOOD CELLS WHICH POSSESS AMINE STORAGE VESICLES AND A CELL
MEMBRANE TRANSPORT MECHANISM ARE:
A. Red blood cells
B. Basophils
C. Eosinophils
D. Lymphocytes
E. Platelets

Ref. 86 - p. 339

184. THE SIMILARITY BETWEEN THE ABOVE BLOOD CELLS AND AMINE-
CONTAINING CELLS IN THE BRAIN MAKES THEM USEFUL IN STUDYING
THE BIOCHEMISTRY OF:
A. Schizophrenia
B. Affective disorders
C. Heroin addiction
D. Alcoholism
E. Epilepsy

Ref. 86 - p. 339

185. IMIPRAMINE TREATMENT IS ASSOCIATED IN THOSE BLOOD CELLS
WHICH HAVE TRANSPORT MECHANISMS FOR BIOGENIC AMINES WITH:
A. Inhibition of biogenic amine transport
B. Destruction of biogenic amine transport
C. Stimulation of biogenic amine transport
D. No immediate effect but delayed stimulation
E. No immediate effect but delayed inhibition

Ref. 86 - p. 341

186. THE EFFECT OF LITHIUM ON THOSE BLOOD CELLS WHICH HAVE
TRANSPORT MECHANISMS FOR BIOGENIC AMINES IS:
A. Similar to that of imipramine
B. Stimulation of serotonin and metaraminol transport
C. Present only when in-vitro preparation is used
D. All of the above
E. None of the above

Ref. 86 - p. 341

187. IN THE TREATMENT OF MANIC-DEPRESSIVE DISEASE WITH LITHIUM
CARBONATE:
A. There is no effect in the acute manic state but subsequent cycles
can be prevented
B. Acute manic and depressive states show an equivalent response
C. Acute manic states respond but acute depressive states do not respond
D. A depression may be precipitated
E. There is a marked placebo effect in depression

Ref. 87 - p. 350

188. THE NUMBER OF POSITIVE RESPONSES TO LITHIUM IS HIGHEST IN:
A. The youngest age group
B. The middle-aged group
C. Those over 60
D. Hysteria
E. Depression

Ref. 87 - p. 348

189. IN THE COMPARISON BETWEEN LITHIUM AND CHLORPROMAZINE FOR TREATMENT OF MANIA:
  A. Lithium appears to be superior
  B. Double-blind study is not meaningful in the true sense of the term
  C. Lithium has a relative lack of unpleasant side effects
  D. All of the above
  E. None of the above   Ref. 88 - p. 352

190. METHYSERGIDE AS A TREATMENT FOR MANIA:
  A. Is based on its antagonism to tryptamine
  B. Is based on its antagonism to serotonin
  C. Has had inconsistent results in the studies
  D. All of the above
  E. None of the above   Ref. 89 - p. 354

191. PATIENTS TREATED WITH L-DOPA SHOW:
  A. Increase in psychosis if schizophrenic
  B. Decreased sleep and REM time
  C. Side effects of hypomania, hypersexuality and suicidal behavior
  D. Decreased dose requirement when peripheral decarboxylase inhibitors are added to the regimen
  E. All of the above   Ref. 90 - p. 361

192. WHEN THYROID HORMONE IS ADMINISTERED WITH IMIPRAMINE TO DEPRESSED PATIENTS:
  A. Clinical antidepressant effects occur more rapidly
  B. Antidepressant effects of imipramine are blocked
  C. There is an increase in leukopenia
  D. No demonstrable improvement occurs
  E. The mixture is contraindicated   Ref. 91 - p. 360

193. PARTICULARLY SENSITIVE TO RELATIVELY LOW DOSES OF MARIJUANA IS:
  A. Selective perception
  B. Immediate recall of preceding thoughts in order to keep on track
  C. Capacity for goal-directed thinking
  D. All of the above
  E. None of the above   Ref. 92 - p. 198

194. MARIJUANA INTOXICATION HAS SIGNIFICANT EFFECTS ON:
  A. Complex reaction time (through impairment of vigilance)
  B. Recent memory, recall and comprehension of written information
  C. Accuracy of time estimation
  D. All of the above
  E. None of the above   Ref. 92 - p. 198

195. TETRAHYDROCANNABINOL (THC) INDUCES:
  A. Euphoria
  B. Depersonalization
  C. Temporal disintegration (confusion of past, present, and future)
  D. All of the above
  E. None of the above   Ref. 93 - p. 210

196. THE EFFECT OF GLUTETHIMIDE, METHYPRYLON, AND PENTOBARBI-
TAL ON SLEEP IS TO:
A. Increase REM sleep
B. Decrease REM sleep
C. Decrease REM sleep on withdrawal of medication
D. Spare REM sleep
E. Increase stage 4 sleep   Ref. 94 - p. 218

197. FOLLOWING WITHDRAWAL OF THE ABOVE DRUGS:
A. There is a decrease of dream frequency
B. Unpleasant dreams and nightmares are reported
C. There is a feeling of having slept well
D. All of the above
E. None of the above   Ref. 94 - p. 216

198. AN EFFECTIVE TREATMENT FOR SLEEPWALKING AND NIGHT TERRORS
WOULD THEORETICALLY BE DRUG-INDUCED SUPPRESSION OF:
A. REM sleep
B. Stage 1
C. Stage 2
D. Stage 4
E. REM rebound   Ref. 95 - p. 224

199. DRUGS WHICH SIGNIFICANTLY SUPPRESS STAGE 4 SLEEP ARE:
A. Flurazepam
B. Glutethimide
C. Pentobarbital
D. Chlordiazepoxide and diazepam
E. All of the above   Ref. 95 - p. 224

200. DRUGS WHICH DO NOT PRODUCE REM SUPPRESSION NOR REM REBOUND
ON WITHDRAWAL:
A. Chloral hydrate
B. Flurazepam
C. Glutethimide
D. Pentobarbital
E. All of the above   Ref. 95 - p. 224

201. THE ABILITY TO TOLERATE ANTIPSYCHOTIC DRUGS SEEMS TO BE
DIRECTLY CORRELATED WITH:
A. Body weight
B. Body type
C. Sex
D. Psychomotor activity
E. Severity of the psychosis   Ref. 96 - p. 190

202. THYROID STIMULATING HORMONE WHEN COMBINED WITH IMIPRAMINE:
A. Does not change the response to imipramine
B. Is contraindicated in combination with imipramine
C. Produces a more rapid response to imipramine
D. Is less effective than triiodothyronine
E. None of the above   Ref. 97 - p. 191

203. A DRUG WHICH IS EFFECTIVE IN THE TREATMENT OF GILLES DE LA TOURETTE'S DISEASE IS:
    A. L-DOPA
    B. Haloperidol
    C. D- amphetamine
    D. Diazepam
    E. Desmethylimipramine   Ref. 98 - p. 204

204. THE EFFECTIVENESS OF THE ABOVE DRUG IN THE TREATMENT OF GILLES DE LA TOURETTE'S DISEASE SUGGESTS THE DISORDER IS DUE TO:
    A. Disorder in the "reward centers" of the hypothalamus
    B. The medial forebrain bundle in the lateral hypothalamus
    C. Hyperactivity of the dopaminergic systems
    D. Markedly reduced levels of dopamine in the corpus striatum
    E. Psychogenic factors   Ref. 98 - p. 204

205. THE CONDITION IN WHICH AN INDIVIDUAL CHOOSES TO LIVE HIS LIFE AS A MEMBER OF THE OPPOSITE SEX IS KNOWN AS:
    A. Inversion
    B. Transvestism
    C. Transsexualism
    D. Intersex
    E. Homosexuality   Ref. 99 - p. 117

206. IF PROFOUND CROSS-GENDER ORIENTATION IS DETECTED EARLY IN LIFE:
    A. Intensive individual psychotherapy is essential
    B. Treatment should be instituted no later than age 5 or 6
    C. Family counseling should be instituted
    D. Therapist should be a person of the same sex as the child
    E. All of the above   Ref. 99 - p. 117

207. THE SUICIDE RATE IN A LARGE CITY WITH A NINE-MONTH NEWS-PAPER BLACKOUT:
    A. Was no different from that period when newspapers were printed
    B. Rose compared to periods when newspapers were printed
    C. Was significantly lower in the female population under 35
    D. Was not related to suggestive effect of printing suicide stories
    E. None of the above   Ref. 100 - p. 148

208. THE SUICIDE RATE IN THE UNITED STATES IS (PER 100,000):
    A. 1.6
    B. 4.8
    C. 10.1
    D. 32.6
    E. 40.5   Ref. 101 - p. 153

209. THE SUICIDE RATE IS HIGHEST IN:
    A. Los Angeles
    B. San Francisco
    C. New York City
    D. Manhattan
    E. London   Ref. 101 - p. 153

210. ALTHOUGH THE ACTUAL NUMBER OF SUICIDES IS AT LEAST 3 OR 4
TIMES HIGHER, THE LATEST STATISTICS LIST (PER YEAR):
   A. 12,000
   B. 18,000
   C. 24,000
   D. 30,000
   E. 36,000   Ref. 102 - p. 158

211. CHARACTERISTIC OF THE SUICIDE-PRONE PERSON IS:
   A. Less involvement in the future and inability to elaborate plans
   B. Physical well-being
   C. Avoidance of alcohol
   D. Being married
   E. None of the above   Ref. 102 - p. 159

212. A SIGNIFICANT DIFFERENCE BETWEEN VIOLENT AND NON-VIOLENT
PRISONERS IS:
   A. Height
   B. Race
   C. Religion
   D. Body-buffer zone
   E. Social background   Ref. 103 - p. 59

213. DSM-II DIFFERS FROM DSM-I IN:
   A. Abolishing the term "reaction" in the case of major psychiatric
      syndromes
   B. Introducing the category "personality pattern disorder"
   C. Putting mental retardation at the end of the classification system
   D. Defining syndrome, symptom, and symptom complex
   E. Having consulted 10% of United States psychiatrists
                                                 Ref. 104 - p. 65

214. THE TERM "POST-PARTUM PSYCHOSIS" IS PRESENT:
   A. Only in DSM-I
   B. Only in DSM-II
   C. In both Diagnostic and Statistical Manuals
   D. In neither manual
   E. The term does not exist   Ref. 104 - p. 70

215. THE TERM "PASSIVE-AGGRESSIVE PERSONALITY DISORDER":
   A. Is found only in DSM-I
   B. Is found only in DSM-II
   C. Is found in both manuals
   D. Is found in neither manual
   E. Does not exist   Ref. 104 - p. 68

216. DSM-II USES AS A BASIS OF TAXONOMY:
   A. Phenomenology
   B. Etiology
   C. Course and prognosis
   D. All of the above
   E. None of the above   Ref. 104 - p. 69

217. THE TERM "NEUROSIS" WAS INTRODUCED BY:
A. Freud
B. Janet
C. Kraepelin
D. Bleuler
E. Cullen   Ref. 105 - p. 80

218. THE "MAUVE FACTOR" IS:
A. Essential factor in tissue culture media
B. Found in the corpus striatum in parkinsonism
C. Reported to be a chromatographic finding in the urine of schizophrenics
D. Produced by massive doses of phenothiazines
E. A catecholamine   Ref. 106 - p. 90

219. TREATMENT OF SCHIZOPHRENIA WITH NIACINAMIDE:
A. Is more successful in early infantile autism
B. Has not been found to be effective in certain controlled studies
C. Is now an accepted form of treatment
D. All of the above
E. None of the above   Ref. 106 - p. 92

220. A FOUR-YEAR FOLLOW-UP ON THE PATIENTS OF GRINKER'S BORDER-
LINE SYNDROME REVEALED THE FOLLOWING, EXCEPT:
A. There was evidence in social functioning of movement to schizophrenia
B. Adaptations are made within very narrow constricted limits
C. There is a steady employment picture
D. Very few human object relations in their lives
E. Little individual change in their social functioning
                    Ref. 107 - p. 7

221. IN THE FAMILIES OF CHILDREN WITH DEPRESSIONS THERE IS A HIGH
INCIDENCE OF:
A. Parental depression
B. Parental aggression and hostility directed to the child
C. Overt parental rejection
D. All of the above
E. None of the above   Ref. 108 - p. 14

222. DEPRESSIVE SYMPTOMATOLOGY IN CHILDREN INCLUDE THE
FOLLOWING, EXCEPT:
A. Sad appearance
B. Absence of auto-erotic activities
C. Withdrawal
D. Expression of feelings of being unloved
E. Insomnia   Ref. 108 - p. 12

223. THE MOST FREQUENT SYMPTOM WHICH LEADS TO PSYCHIATRIC
REFERRAL OF THE DEPRESSED CHILD IS:
A. Failure to thrive
B. Overt aggressive behavior
C. Expressed feelings of unhappiness and being unloved
D. Developmental retardation
E. Loss of weight   Ref. 108 - p. 13

224. THE INTEGRATION OF GERIATRIC PATIENTS WITH YOUNGER
PATIENTS IN A PSYCHIATRIC HOSPITAL GENERALLY LEADS TO:
A. Physical harm and abuse from younger patients
B. Defensive withdrawal on the part of the elderly patients
C. Greater confusion in those patients who were impaired in cognitive
functioning
D. Greater tolerance of deviant behavior in the elderly, such as occasional
incontinence
E. Uninvolvement on the part of the younger patients with the elderly weaker
patients   Ref. 109 - p. 28

225. DEPRESSED PATIENTS GENERALLY HAVE THE FOLLOWING ABNOR-
MALITIES IN THEIR SLEEP PATTERN, EXCEPT FOR:
A. Reduction in delta sleep (stages 3 and 4)
B. Decreased nonrapid eye movement sleep (NREM sleep) with increased
awakenings
C. Lengthened REM latencies (amount of time asleep until the onset of the
first REM period)
D. Usually decreased REM sleep, with occasional marked elevation of
REM time
E. Increase in REM and NREM sleep with recovery from illness
Ref. 110 - p. 39

226. THE SLEEP PATTERN IN MANIA TENDS TO BE:
A. Reduction in total sleep and marked decrease in REM sleep
B. Similar to that in depression except for increase in delta sleep
C. Opposite to the findings in depression
D. Impossible to record with accuracy
E. None of the above   Ref. 110 - p. 39

227. THE EFFECT OF LITHIUM CARBONATE ON THE SLEEP PATTERN IN
MANIA IS TO:
A. Increase REM sleep
B. Increase delta sleep time
C. Lower total sleep time
D. Markedly increase sleep latency (sleep onset difficulty)
E. Lower delta sleep time   Ref. 110 - p. 39

228. REM SLEEP IS SUPPRESSED TO SOME DEGREE BY:
A. Barbiturates
B. Iminodibenzyl derivatives
C. MAO inhibitors
D. Lithium
E. All of the above   Ref. 110 - p. 39

229. A DRUG WHICH APPEARS TO INCREASE DELTA SLEEP TIME IN MANIC-
DEPRESSIVE PATIENTS IS:
A. Pentobarbital
B. Chlorpromazine
C. Lithium
D. Imipramine
E. Isocarboxazid   Ref. 110 - p. 39

230. THE PSYCHIATRIC STATUS SCHEDULE (PSS) IS AN INSTRUMENT
DESIGNED FOR EVALUATION OF PSYCHOPATHOLOGY AND:
A. Impairment in formal role functioning
B. Impairment in conduct of leisure time and daily routine
C. Impairment in personal relationships
D. All of the above
E. None of the above   Ref. 111 - p. 55

231. AN ADVANTAGE OF THE PSYCHIATRIC STATUS SCHEDULE IS:
A. It is relevant for non-patients and out-patients, as well as in-patients
B. Administration, interview, and evaluation are completed simultaneously
C. Interviewer need not be a mental health professional
D. Evaluation takes from 30 to 50 minutes
E. All of the above   Ref. 111 - p. 42

232. HIGH ANTI-CNS ANTIBODY TITERS HAVE BEEN FOUND IN:
A. Patients with chronic brain syndrome
B. Schizrenia
C. Neurosis
D. All of the above
E. None of the above   Ref. 112 - p. 64

233. THE ADDED ANTICHOLINERGIC ACTION OF ANTIPARKINSONIAN DRUGS
IN PHENOTHIAZINE THERAPY INCREASES THE DANGER OF THE DE-
VELOPMENT OF:
A. Agranulocytosis
B. Heat stroke
C. Photosensitivity
D. Dystonia
E. Jaundice   Ref. 113 - p. 1787

234. THE ABOVE DANGER OCCURS BECAUSE OF THE EFFECT OF
PHENOTHIAZINES ON:
A. Hypothalamus
B. Ascending reticular system
C. Liver
D. Reticuloendothelial system
E. Corpus striatum   Ref. 113 - p. 1787

235. THE MARIJUANA-SMOKING COLLEGE STUDENT:
A. Is more likely to be at the top of his class
B. Describes himself as less moody and happier than nonsmokers
C. Represents a majority of college students
D. All of the above
E. None of the above   Ref. 114 - p. 1749

236. DEMONSTRATORS WHO WERE ARRESTED AT THE DEMOCRATIC
NATIONAL CONVENTION IN CHICAGO IN 1968:
A. Came mainly from lower class origins
B. Tended to express beliefs in violence when necessary
C. May best be understood in terms of a youth culture
D. Protested against the Democratic party
E. Were dropouts   Ref. 115 - p. 1759

40

237. DURING INTOXICATION, ALCOHOLICS:
A. Become more cooperative and friendly
B. Will generally stop drinking when they have had enough
C. Become markedly regressed and lose controls
D. Recall vividly the events which occur
E. Become more euphoric than anticipated before drinking began
Ref. 116 - p. 1702

238. ALCOHOLICS DO NOT PREDICT THAT DURING INTOXICATION THEY WILL:
A. Become more sociable
B. Be more aggressive, openly sexual, and dysphoric
C. Experience amnesia
D. All of the above
E. None of the above
Ref. 116 - p. 1697

239. THE COMPREHENSIVE HEALTH PLANNING LEGISLATION, PUBLIC LAW 89-749 IS ALSO KNOWN AS:
A. Medicare
B. Medicaid
C. MIC Project
D. Partnership for Health
E. Action for Mental Health
Ref. 117 - p. 1725

240. THE PURPOSE OF PUBLIC LAW 89-749 IS TO:
A. Involve the community in the development of a health program
B. Draw on community leaders for mental hygiene programs
C. Aid the elderly and indigent to obtain medical treatment
D. Gradually phase out state hospital system
E. Replace OEO Neighborhood Health Centers
Ref. 117 - p. 1725

241. TITLE 18 AND TITLE 19 OF THE SOCIAL SECURITY AMENDMENTS OF 1965 ARE:
A. Medicare and Medicaid
B. Medicaid and Medicare
C. Maternal and Infant Care Projects and OEO Neighborhood Health Centers
D. OEO Neighborhood Health Centers and Maternal and Infant Care Projects
E. Regional Medical Program and Partnership for Health
Ref. 117 - p. 1724

242. THE FOLLOWING NAMES ARE ASSOCIATED WITH THE STUDY OF CURRENT PROBLEMS OF YOUTH, EXCEPT:
A. Kenneth Keniston
B. Julius Axelrod
C. Peter Blos
D. Erik Erikson
E. Anna Freud
Ref. 118 - p. 1742

243. DRIVE-DEFENSE CONSTELLATIONS IN COLLEGE STUDENT PATIENTS
WHICH CURRENTLY RECEIVE CONSIDERABLE ENVIRONMENTAL
STIMULATION AND REINFORCEMENT INCLUDE:
A. Regression (in object relations, use of drugs)
B. Rebellion
C. Dislocation (sense of loss of involvement)
D. All of the above
E. None of the above   Ref. 118 - p. 1737

244. ODORS ARE FREQUENTLY REPORTED AS PRECIPITANTS OF ATTACKS
OF:
A. Ulcerative colitis
B. Duodenal ulcer
C. Migraine
D. Asthma
E. Neurodermatitis   Ref. 119 - p. 486

245. THE ABOVE ODORS CAN BE CLASSIFIED OPERATIONALLY IN THE
CATEGORY OF:
A. Food or oral odors
B. Cleanliness-uncleanliness or anal odors
C. Romance or genital odors
D. All of the above
E. None of the above   Ref. 119 - p. 486

246. IN A CONDITIONING EXPERIMENT TO THE WORD "COW", REINFORCED
WITH AN ELECTRIC SHOCK, AND HEART RATE RECORDED BY A
CARDIOTACHOMETER:
A. The electric shock is the conditional stimulus
B. The word "cow" is the conditional stimulus
C. The word "cow" is the unconditional stimulus
D. The heart rate is the conditional stimulus
E. None of the above   Ref. 119 - p. 484

247. THE SPREAD OF ANXIETY TO WORDS RELATED TO THE CONDITIONED
STIMULUS:
A. Is greater at the aware than the unaware level
B. Is greater at the unaware than the aware level
C. Is unrelated to awareness or unawareness
D. There is no spread of anxiety to related words
E. Awareness increases generalization to related words
                                        Ref. 119 - p. 485

248. THE PERCENTAGE OF STAGE 4 SLEEP IN PREPUBERTAL CHILDREN
DIAGNOSED AS BEING PSYCHOTIC:
A. Is twice that of normal children
B. Is not different from that observed in normal children
C. Is not influenced by the presence of brain damage
D. Is similar to that seen in adult schizophrenics
E. Is lower than that seen in adult schizophrenics
                                        Ref. 120 - p. 502

42

249. THE FOLLOWING IS CHARACTERISTIC OF THE USE OF PORNOGRAPHY, EXCEPT:
    A. It is not a perversion
    B. It must be suited to the personal style and needs of the user
    C. Voyeurism is a component
    D. Sadism and masochism are components
    E. There is always a victim   Ref. 121 - p. 490

250. WHAT MAY BE DESCRIBED AS THE PORNOGRAPHY OF WOMEN:
    A. Does not exist
    B. May be found in fashion magazine photographs
    C. Appears in certain types of romance stories
    D. Will also tend to excite men
    E. Are photographs of nude men   Ref. 121 - p. 499

251. THE PORNOGRAPHY OF AN INDIVIDUAL IS RELEVANT BECAUSE:
    A. It contains latently the historical origins of his perversion
    B. It contains latently the fantasy elaborations of his perversion
    C. Successful pornography is not idiosyncratic, and therefore extracts features that the audience shares in common
    D. All of the above
    E. None of the above   Ref. 121 - p. 496

252. PORNOGRAPHY IS CHARACTERIZED BY:
    A. Induction of genital excitement in an observer
    B. Being a daydream which is usually but not necessarily overtly sexual
    C. Being projected into written or pictorial material
    D. Requiring an observer's fantasies to be added
    E. All of the above   Ref. 121 - p. 490

253. MULTIPROBLEM FAMILIES TEND TO BE CHARACTERIZED BY THE FOLLOWING, EXCEPT:
    A. Irony, sarcasm, and laughter
    B. Few verbal attempts at limit setting
    C. Disagree more than they agree
    D. Much potential for explosive behavior
    E. Highly assertive and unfriendly   Ref. 122 - p. 532

254. CONSTRICTED FAMILIES TEND TO BE CHARACTERIZED BY THE FOLLOWING, EXCEPT:
    A. Extreme clarity in speech patterns
    B. Much parental limit setting
    C. Little agreement or disagreement
    D. Inhibition of affective expression and spontaneity
    E. One scapegoat in the family   Ref. 122 - p. 533

255. FAMILIES WITH OFFICIAL CHILD-LABELED PROBLEMS TEND TO BE CHARACTERIZED BY THE FOLLOWING, EXCEPT:
    A. Low-keyed, sullen, non-cooperative atmosphere
    B. Considerable show of limit setting
    C. Signs of one scapegoat in the family
    D. Clear, non-fragmented speech patterns
    E. Absence of mutual attacks   Ref. 122 - p. 534

256. "NORMAL" FAMILIES TEND TO BE CHARACTERIZED BY THE
FOLLOWING, EXCEPT:
A. Tendency to stay on the same topic
B. Display of a wide range of intensity of feelings
C. High task commitment
D. Friendly and supportive atmosphere with respect for differences
E. Very little intrusiveness   Ref. 122 - p. 566

257. THE COST OF BEING MAINTAINED ON CHRONIC HEMODIALYSIS FOR
KIDNEY FAILURE IS:
A. Lower in home dialysis compared to hospital dialysis
B. Beyond the reach of most patients who require it
C. At least $10,000 per year
D. All of the above
E. None of the above   Ref. 123 - p. 566

258. A FREQUENTLY NOTED DEFENSE MECHANISM IN PATIENTS ON
CHRONIC HEMODIALYSIS IS:
A. Denial
B. Sublimation
C. Repression
D. Reaction formation
E. Anticipation   Ref. 123 - p. 573

259. THE MOTORCYCLE SYNDROME INCLUDES THE FOLLOWING SYMPTOMS,
EXCEPT:
A. History of accident-proneness extending to early childhood
B. Distant relationship with father, strong identification with mother
C. Active and competitive striving
D. Poor impulse control
E. Unusual preoccupation with the motorcycle
          Ref. 124 - p. 1595

260. THE MOTORCYCLE SYNDROME:
A. May be specific to accident-prone cyclists
B. When recognized early enough should receive the indicated treatment
which may significantly lower the increasing number of accidents
C. May provide clues to the understanding of accident-prone drivers of
automobiles
D. All of the above
E. None of the above   Ref. 124 - p. 1594

261. THE TREATMENT OF WOMEN WHO ARE TRANSSEXUAL WITH TES-
TOSTERONE LEADS TO:
A. Hirsutism without development of acne
B. Protuberant phallus
C. Cessation of menses
D. Appreciable diminution of breast size
E. No change in voice   Ref. 125 - p. 1599

262. THE TREATMENT OF MEN WHO ARE TRANSSEXUAL WITH ESTROGENS
LEADS TO:
A. Diminished libido and impotence
B. Rise in the pitch of the voice
C. Removal of the beard
D. Ideal female body proportions
E. Increased libido   Ref. 125 - p. 1599

44

263.   FIRST-BORN CHILDREN ARE MORE LIKELY TO BE:
A.   Participants in dangerous sports, but more frightened of injury
B.   Offering to participate in situations involving bodily risk only after
      others have volunteered
C.   Less self-confident in a group, but often group leaders
D.   All of the above
E.   None of the above   Ref. 126 - p. 1608

264.   AT A MILITARY RECRUIT TRAINING CAMP, ONLY CHILDREN WOULD
       BE MORE LIKELY THAN FIRST CHILDREN TO:
A.   Consult the psychiatrist
B.   Be diagnosed as psychoneurotic
C.   Be discharged from the service
D.   All of the above
E.   None of the above   Ref. 126 - p. 1604

DIRECTIONS FOR QUESTIONS 265 THROUGH 270:

FOR EACH NUMBERED WORD OR STATEMENT SELECT THE LETTERED
STATEMENT THAT IS MOST CLOSELY ASSOCIATED WITH IT:

A.   Primary prevention of mental illness
B.   Secondary prevention of mental illness
C.   Tertiary prevention of mental illness
D.   All of the above
E.   None of the above

265. ___   Social psychiatric care aimed at reducing impairment or curing the
           illness
266. ___   Community psychiatry
267. ___   Marijuana use
268. ___   Prevention of appearance of diseases
269. ___   Melioration of disease at an early stage
270. ___   Battered child syndrome   Ref. 127 - p. 1622

FOR EACH OF THE FOLLOWING MULTIPLE CHOICE QUESTIONS
SELECT THE MOST APPROPRIATE ANSWER:

271.   A COMPARISON IN THE PATIENT POPULATION SEEN IN PSYCHIATRIC
       EMERGENCY IN A GENERAL HOSPITAL EMERGENCY SERVICE IN THE
       LATE 1950'S VERSUS THE LATE 1960'S REVEALS:
A.   Striking shift to a younger age group being treated
B.   Striking increase in rate of referral to inpatient care
C.   Decrease in patient load relative to the increase in the area population
D.   Increase in the over 65-category
E.   Under-utilization of the facility   Ref. 128 - p. 1628

272.   THE COMMUNITY MENTAL HEALTH CENTERS ACT OF 1963 (PUBLIC
       LAW 88-164):
A.   Defines the therapeutic aims of community psychiatry
B.   Encourages family therapy as a primary therapeutic modality
C.   Requires an emergency facility as an integral part of every community
      health center
D.   Requires establishment of methadone maintenance clinics as a part
      of a community health center
E.   Requires that a patient receive psychiatric care within his community
                                           Ref. 128 - p. 1631

273. SUICIDAL BEHAVIOR IS PARTICULARLY LIKELY TO OCCUR WHEN:
    A. There is hostility and death wishes from the family and other signifi-
       cant external objects
    B. The suicidal person is unable to retaliate
    C. External support is unavailable or withdrawn
    D. All of the above
    E. None of the above   Ref. 129 - p. 1654

274. THE LEAST SEVERE CATEGORY OF CHARACTERISTIC FORMAL SIGNS
    OF SCHIZOPHRENIC THOUGHT DISORDER IS:
    A. Circumstantiality and concreteness
    B. Autistic intrusions
    C. Perseverations, blocking and neologisms
    D. Predicative identification
    E. Loosening of associations   Ref. 130 - p. 1657

275. THE MOST SEVERE CATEGORY OF CHARACTERISTIC FORMAL SIGNS
    OF SCHIZOPHRENIC THOUGHT DISORDER IS:
    A. Circumstantiality and concreteness
    B. Autistic intrusions and loosening of associations
    C. Perseverations, blocking and neologisms
    D. Predicative identifications
    E. Loosening of associations   Ref. 130 - p. 1657

276. A CLINICAL FEATURE THAT IS PATHOGNOMONIC OF SCHIZOPHRENIA
    IS:
    A. Characteristic disturbance of thinking
    B. Flattening of affect
    C. Delusions and hallucinations
    D. All of the above
    E. None of the above   Ref. 130 - p. 1655

277. THE XYY MALE IS:
    A. Not found in the Negro race
    B. Always of subnormal intelligence
    C. Several inches taller than the average male
    D. Found to have an abnormal EEG
    E. Invariably associated with aggressive behavior
                                            Ref. 131 - p. 1661

278. THE FOLLOWING IS TRUE OF THE XYY COMBINATION, EXCEPT:
    A. Unipolar affective disorder is more common
    B. The combination occurs in not less than one in every 500 male births
    C. About 200,000 XYY males live in the United States
    D. The frequency of antisocial behavior and crime may not be greater
       than that of the average citizen
    E. Height averages six inches more than the average male
                                            Ref. 131 - p. 1662

279. SMALL DOSES OF TRIIODOTHYRONINE ARE OF VALUE IN THE TREAT-
MENT OF DEPRESSION:
   A. When combined with tricyclic antidepressants because of the poten-
tiation of the antidepressant effect
   B. Since most depressives tend to be mildly hypothyroid
   C. To prevent relapse following a favorable response to antidepressant
medication
   D. In the involutional period
   E. But are contraindicated when protriptyline is used because of the danger
of precipitating a hypertensive crisis
                                             Ref. 132 - p. 1668

280. TRIIODOTHYRONINE ADMINISTERED WITH IMIPRAMINE:
   A. Enhances the effectiveness of imipramine
   B. Delays response to imipramine
   C. Is less effective in women
   D. Is contraindicated
   E. None of the above   Ref. 132 - p. 1669

281. THERE IS A SIGNIFICANTLY HIGHER PROPORTION OF UNSUCCESSFUL
DISCHARGE FROM A METHADONE MAINTENANCE PROGRAM WHEN:
   A. Patients receive a six week hospitalization for methadone stabilization
prior to out-patient maintenance
   B. Maintained on methadone in amount less than 80 mg
   C. Patients reside with their families
   D. There is work at which the patient is employed
   E. The patient has been in the program more than one year
                                             Ref. 133 - p. 1393

282. THE FOLLOWING IS TRUE OF PATIENTS ON METHADONE MAINTENANCE
PROGRAM FOLLOW-UP, EXCEPT:
   A. Most of the patients continue to use heroin
   B. More are employed than before methadone
   C. Fewer are involved with the law
   D. Few stop taking methadone
   E. Some continue to use other drugs regularly
                                             Ref. 133 - p. 1392

283. THE TERM "NEURASTHENIA":
   A. Is no longer used in current diagnostic systems
   B. Was originated in Europe
   C. Implies that the person suffers from easy fatigability and chronic
weakness
   D. Should not be used as a diagnosis since it does not appear in DSM-II
   E. Was first used by Kraepelin   Ref. 134 - p. 1404

284. THE KILLING OF A NEWBORN BABY (NEONATICIDE):
   A. Is more frequently committed by the mother than by the father
   B. Occurs more often in situations where the mother is married rather
than unmarried
   C. Occurs more often when the mother is over 35 rather than under 35
   D. Is more frequently committed by the father
   E. Is legally distinct from murder in the United States
                                             Ref. 135 - p. 1419

285. THE AIRLIE HOUSE CONFERENCE LED TO:
    A. The new constitution of the American Psychiatric Association
    B. Joint Commission on Mental Health of Children
    C. Action for Mental Health
    D. Medicare
    E. Medicaid
                                        Ref. 136 - p. 1490

286. NEW CAREERS PROGRAMS IN MENTAL HEALTH CAN BE DEVELOPED
    BY:
    A. Radical change
    B. Redesign of systems
    C. Reform of systems
    D. All of the above
    E. None of the above
                                        Ref. 137 - p. 1484

287. IN THE DEVELOPMENT OF A HUMAN RELATIONS TRAINING PROGRAM
    FOR POLICE:
    A. Individual sessions with the policeman and a psychiatrist have proven
       most effective
    B. Training a cadre of policemen in group process techniques is the key
       to an ongoing program
    C. The lecture approach effectively imparts key information enabling
       attitudinal change
    D. Emphasis should not be placed on police-minority group relations
    E. There is little place for the psychiatric consultant
                                        Ref. 138 - p. 1421

288. THE INSULATED CASELOAD IN A NEIGHBORHOOD MENTAL HEALTH
    CENTER:
    A. Is more effective for the middle class patient
    B. Matches the needs of the community rather than matching existing
       services
    C. Involves fewer stress-producing situations for the staff than the
       traditional psychiatric clinic caseload
    D. Is unsuccessful in a poor neighborhood
    E. Leads to an excessive rate of staff turnover
                                        Ref. 139 - p. 1433

289. MENTAL HEALTH PROGRAMS IN THE GHETTO REQUIRE ALL OF THE
    FOLLOWING, EXCEPT:
    A. Centralization of services
    B. New careers concept
    C. Integration with other human services
    D. Vocational training
    E. Community outreach
                                        Ref. 140 - p. 1464

290. THE SIX-MONTH PROGRAM USED TO TRAIN AREA RESIDENTS WITHOUT
    ACADEMIC CREDENTIALS TO BECOME PRIMARY THERAPISTS IN
    GHETTO MENTAL HEALTH CLINICS INCLUDES THE FOLLOWING,
    EXCEPT:
    A. Didactic curriculum
    B. Development of group process
    C. World literature, including American black literature seminars
    D. Sessions on silence, posture, and gesture
    E. Sessions on use of psychotropic medication
                                        Ref. 141-- p. 1475

291. URINARY EXCRETION OF ADENOSINE 3', 5'-MONOPHOSPHATE (CYCLIC AMP) IS:
    A. Higher in manic patients
    B. Lower in depressed patients
    C. Still lower in severely depressed patients
    D. All of the above
    E. None of the above   Ref. 142 - p. 1493

292. THE RICHMOND FELLOWSHIP EXPERIMENT IS:
    A. Designed to improve relations between the United States and England
    B. An outgrowth of the Comprehensive Health Planning legislation
    C. A half-way house
    D. A totally egalitarian community
    E. A failure   Ref. 143 - p. 1500

293. THE TIME OF PEAK SEEKING OF PSYCHIATRIC HELP IN WALK-IN CLINIC AND EMERGENCY ROOM IS:
    A. During menstruation
    B. At midcycle
    C. During premenstruum
    D. All of the above
    E. None of the above   Ref. 144 - p. 1504

294. THE AMOUNT OF TIME DEVOTED TO SLEEP DURING THE SUMMER MONTHS AT THE SOUTH POLE IS:
    A. More than that devoted to sleep in the temperate zone
    B. Less than that in the temperate zone
    C. Similar to that in the temperate zone
    D. More than that seen during the summer months north of the Arctic Circle
    E. Less than that of the Arctic Circle   Ref. 145 - p. 389

295. INCREASES IN PLASMA ACTIVITY OF THE ENZYME CREATINE KINASE OCCUR IN:
    A. Duchenne muscular dystrophy
    B. Acutely psychotic patients of all diagnostic types
    C. The state following physical exercise in athletically untrained individuals
    D. All of the above
    E. None of the above   Ref. 146 - p. 390

296. EVIDENCE FOR A MYOPATHIC PROCESS IN ACUTELY PSYCHOTIC PATIENTS:
    A. Is based on increased creatine kinase activity at the early phase of the psychosis
    B. Is based on the larger response in such patients to exercise of creatine kinase activity
    C. Is found in microscopic studies of muscle biopsy
    D. All of the above
    E. None of the above   Ref. 146 - p. 395

297. AN ADDITIONAL ABNORMALITY WHICH CORRELATES WELL WITH INCREASED ACTIVITY OF CREATINE KINASE IN ACUTELY PSYCHOTIC PATIENTS IS:
   A. Low REM time
   B. High REM time
   C. Increased levels of SGOT and LDH
   D. Prolonged sleep
   E. Decreased levels of SGOT and LDH   Ref. 147 - p. 404

298. JUST BEFORE THE ONSET OF DELIRIUM TREMENS, REM STAGE APPROACHES:
   A. 10% of sleep
   B. 20% of sleep
   C. 50% of sleep
   D. 80% of sleep
   E. 100% of sleep   Ref. 148 - p. 406

299. ALCOHOL INTAKE LEADS TO:
   A. Long latencies for sleep onset
   B. Few awakenings
   C. Increase in REM
   D. Increase in REM sleep
   E. Few changes from one sleep stage to another
                                 Ref. 148 - p. 417

300. SUBJECTS WHO ARE ALCOHOLICS AND WHO ARE ALLOWED HIGH INTAKE OF ALCOHOL IN A LABORATORY WARD SETTING:
   A. Do not taper off their drinking before withdrawal is imposed on them
   B. Have a high incidence of withdrawal phenomena similar to that experienced in their normal environment
   C. Socialize with fellow patients
   D. Have motor impairment and ataxia at the 200 mg/100 cc level
   E. Appear more anxious and depressed after a few hours of drinking although they drink to avoid these symptoms
                                 Ref. 149 - p. 430

301. INFANTILE AUTISM IS CHARACTERIZED BY THE FOLLOWING, EXCEPT:
   A. Profound withdrawal
   B. May not be evident until prepuberty
   C. Obsessive desire for sameness
   D. Mutism or language which has a peculiar use of pronouns, neologisms, and metaphors
   E. Retention of intelligence   Ref. 150 - p. 431

302. CHILDHOOD SCHIZOPHRENIA IS CHARACTERIZED BY THE FOLLOWING, EXCEPT:
   A. It is a heterogeneous group of syndromes including but not restricted to infantile autism
   B. Autistic, withdrawn, and atypical behavior
   C. Failure to develop identity separate from the mother's
   D. Gross immaturity and inadequacy in development
   E. Mental retardation   Ref. 150 - p. 431

303. CHILDHOOD SCHIZOPHRENIA CONSISTS OF:
    A. Infantile autism which excludes organicity and is characterized by early onset
    B. Psychotic disorders which include some features of infantile autism but have an onset later in childhood
    C. Psychotic disorders complicated by an organicity which is demonstrable
    D. All of the above
    E. None of the above   Ref. 150 - p. 432

304. IN CHILDHOOD SCHIZOPHRENIA:
    A. Females outnumber males
    B. The prevalence rate approaches that of adult schizophrenia
    C. There is a high incidence of first born children
    D. Abnormal EEG in seen in nearly all patients
    E. None of the above   Ref. 150 - p. 437

305. INFANTILE AUTISM IS:
    A. Set apart from the rest of childhood schizophrenia in the level of parental education
    B. Associated with abnormalities of the EEG
    C. More frequent in girls
    D. The most common form of childhood schizophrenia
    E. All of the above   Ref. 150 - p. 437

306. IN WOMEN THE NEED TO BE HELD:
    A. Is so compelling in some that it resembles an addiction
    B. Is affected by depression, anxiety, and anger
    C. May be camouflaged with the veil of "adult" sexuality
    D. May be an end in itself
    E. All of the above   Ref. 151 - p. 453

307. IN THE ELDERLY, DECLINE IN PERFORMANCE ABILITIES IS ASSOCIATED CHIEFLY WITH:
    A. Diffuse slowing in the left anterior temporal EEG tracing
    B. Reduction of blood flow in the left parietal cortex
    C. Sociocultural background
    D. All of the above
    E. None of the above   Ref. 152 - p. 1211

308. IN THE ELDERLY, DECLINE IN VERBAL ABILITIES IS ASSOCIATED CHIEFLY WITH:
    A. Focal disturbances in the left anterior temporal EEG
    B. Diffuse slowing in the occipital rhythm
    C. Reduction of blood flow in the left parietal cortex
    D. All of the above
    E. None of the above   Ref. 152 - p. 1211

309. THE SLEEP PATTERNS IN ACUTE SCHIZOPHRENIA DEMONSTRATE:
    A. Unusually prominent amount of REM sleep just before psychotic exacerbation
    B. High increase in REM during the waxing phase
    C. Decrease in REM during the waning phase
    D. Few disruptions in sleep during the waxing phase
    E. None of the above   Ref. 153 - p. 1221

310. ACUTE SCHIZOPHRENIC PATIENTS TEND TO DEMONSTRATE THE
FOLLOWING IN THEIR REM SLEEP:
A. Consistent prolongation of REM latency
B. REM intensity unchanged
C. REM percentages uniformly low
D. All of the above
E. None of the above   Ref. 153 - p. 1220

311. PSYCHOTIC DEPRESSED PATIENTS TEND TO SHOW THE FOLLOWING
IN THEIR REM SLEEP:
A. Very short REM latencies
B. Intense REM activity
C. REM percentages varying from far below to far above normal levels
D. All of the above
E. None of the above   Ref. 153 - p. 1220

312. THE EFFECT OF ANXIETY AND ACUTE STRESS ON THE SLEEP
PATTERNS IS IN THE DIRECTION OF:
A. Decreasing REM
B. Increasing REM
C. No change in REM
D. Increase in total sleep
E. None of the above   Ref. 153 - p. 1220

313. FOLLOWING THERAPEUTIC ABORTION, WOMEN WHO ARE SURVEYED:
A. Who report that they feel content and mentally healthy are in the majority
B. Who report that they feel in worse mental health are in the majority
C. Report that they would not make the same decision again for the most
part
D. Provide data which yields conclusive evidence that the procedure is
not psychologically traumatic
E. None of the above   Ref. 154 - p. 1227

314. THE BASIS FOR A THERAPEUTIC ABORTION ON PSYCHIATRIC GROUNDS
REQUIRES THAT:
A. There be a substantial risk that continuation of pregnancy impairs her
mental health to the degree that she would be dangerous to herself
B. Her mental health be impaired to the degree that she would be dangerous
to the person or property of others
C. She would be in need of supervision or restraint
D. All of the above
E. None of the above   Ref. 155 - p. 1231

315. BASIC TO THE VARYING APPROACHES TO THE PATIENT DYING OF
CANCER IS:
A. That the patient know the full truth
B. Discouragement of denial
C. Support of the patient's denial
D. To avoid discussion of illness or dying with the patient
E. Family therapy   Ref. 156 - p. 1242

52

316. THE DECISION OF A LIVING, GENETICALLY RELATED KIDNEY DONOR
TO DONATE HIS KIDNEY FOR HOMOTRANSPLANTATION TENDS TO BE:
A. Made after prolonged discussions with medical personnel
B. Made immediately
C. Made following acquisition of data required for an informed consent
D. Initially negative, later being changed to a consent
E. Initially positive, later being changed to a refusal
Ref. 157 - p. 1247

317. KIDNEY DONORS TEND TO REGARD THEIR ACT:
A. With regret following the initial enthusiasm
B. As the most meaningful experience of their lives
C. With the detachment and feelings of depersonalization
D. All of the above
E. None of the above
Ref. 157 - p. 1249

318. CRITERIA FOR DETERMINING DEATH INCLUDE:
A. No reflexes
B. No spontaneous respirations
C. Flat, isoelectric EEG
D. All of the above
E. None of the above
Ref. 158 - p. 1255

319. ADDICTS TREATED WITH CYCLAZOCINE ARE MORE LIKELY TO
REMAIN ABSTINENT FROM NARCOTIC USE WHEN:
A. There is a stable heterosexual relationship
B. High motivation exists
C. There is no previous history of illegal activity
D. With the concomitant use of methadone, heroin effect is blocked
E. They are under parental supervision
Ref. 159 - p. 1259

320. MATERNAL PREMEDICATION HAS THE FOLLOWING EFFECT ON THE
NEONATE'S CONDITION, EXCEPT:
A. EEG alteration
B. Sucking behavior
C. Lag in adaptation to breast feeding
D. Low Apgar score
E. Subtle effects on mother-neonate interaction
Ref. 160 - p. 1264

321. THE DAY HOSPITAL WITH SHORT-TERM INTENSIVE TREATMENT IS
SUITABLE FOR:
A. The acute patient
B. The chronic patient
C. The heroin addict
D. All of the above
E. None of the above
Ref. 161 - p. 1273

322. ULLMAN HAS INVESTIGATED IN DREAMS ELICITED DURING REM SLEEP
AND THEIR ASSOCIATIONS THE EFFECTS OF:
A. Psychotic states
B. Epilepsy
C. Extrasensory phenomena
D. Tranquilizer and anti-depressant medication
E. Psychotherapy
Ref. 162 - p. 1288

53

323. THE USE OF HIGH DOSES OF NICOTINIC ACID AND NICOTINAMIDE IN
THE TREATMENT OF SCHIZOPHRENIA IS:
A. Inadvisable in women during pregnancy
B. To be used with caution in patients with a history of ulcer, gout,
diabetes, or liver disease
C. Based on a postulated defect in the transmethylation of nor-epinephrine
to epinephrine
D. All of the above
E. None of the above   Ref. 163 - p. 1290

324. THE USE OF NIACIN IN THE DOSES WHICH HAVE BEEN RECOMMENDED
BY SOME INVESTIGATORS FOR THE TREATMENT OF SCHIZOPHRENIA:
A. Is below a maximum of 3 gm/day
B. Causes a significant rise in serum cholesterol
C. Causes a significant drop in serum uric acid levels
D. Has no effect on liver function tests
E. Causes hyperglycemia in nondiabetics
Ref. 163 - p. 1293

325. A TOXIC PSYCHOSIS WITH PARANOID AND HALLUCINATORY SYMPTOMS
MAY DEVELOP FOLLOWING INGESTION OF THE CONTENTS OF:
A. Benzedrex inhaler
B. Wyamine inhaler
C. Dristan inhaler (post-1966 variety)
D. All of the above
E. None of the above   Ref. 164 - p. 1315

326. THE ACTIVE INGREDIENT IN THE ABOVE INHALERS IS:
A. Benzedrine
B. Amphetamine
C. Methamphetamine
D. Propylhexedrine
E. Mephentermine   Ref. 164 - p. 1315

327. COMPUTER DERIVED GLOBAL JUDGMENT (CGJ) IS A TECHNIQUE
APPLYING SEQUENTIAL ANALYSIS TO YIELD COMPUTER DECISIONS
THAT PATIENTS ARE:
A. Significantly better
B. Worse
C. Unchanged
D. All of the above
E. None of the above   Ref. 165 - p. 1057

328. THE DATA FOR THE GLOBAL DECISIONS IN THE ABOVE COMPUTER
TECHNIQUE ARE SIX SMOOTHED BEHAVIOR FACTOR SCORES AMONG
WHICH IS NOT INCLUDED:
A. Acceptable behavior
B. Paranoia
C. Disorganization
D. Depression
E. Antisocial behavior   Ref. 165 - p. 1058

329. MARKED ELEVATIONS OF URINARY CORTICOSTEROID EXCRETION
      OCCUR IN SCHIZOPHRENIC EPISODES DURING THE STAGE OF:
      A. Recovery
      B. Acute psychotic turmoil
      C. Psychotic ego reintegration
      D   "Parasitic" phase
      E. "Compliant" phase   Ref. 166 - p. 1078

330. THE PHASE OF ORGANIZED PSYCHOSIS:
      A. Is similar endocrinologically but not psychologically to the stage of
          ego disintegration
      B. Is similar endocrinologically and psychologically to the stage of ego
          disintegration
      C. Is dissimilar endocrinologically and psychologically from the stage
          of ego disintegration
      D. Is similar endocrinologically and psychologically to the recovery stage
      E. Is dissimilar endocrinologically and psychologically to the recovery
          stage   Ref. 166 - p. 1076

      DIRECTIONS FOR QUESTIONS 331 THROUGH 336:

      FOR EACH NUMBERED WORD OR STATEMENT SELECT THE LETTERED
      STATEMENT THAT IS MOST CLOSELY ASSOCIATED WITH IT:

      A. Acute psychotic turmoil, or severe ego disintegration
      B. Psychotic ego reintegration, or psychotic equilibrium
      C. "Anaclitic" depression
      D. Recovery
      E. "Parasitic" and "compliant" stages

331. ___ Loss of a sense of identity
332. ___ Prominent sense of loneliness and devalued self-image
333. ___ Dependency upon others without having passed through psychotic ego
          organization stage
334. ___ Delusional system becomes of primary interest
335. ___ Severe annihilation anxiety, fears of imminent death, and fantasies
          of world destruction
336. ___ Development of omnipotent sense of identity
                                               Ref. 166 - pp. 1069,1070

      FOR EACH OF THE FOLLOWING MULTIPLE CHOICE QUESTIONS
      SELECT THE MOST APPROPRIATE ANSWER:

337. THE REINFORCING POTENCY OF ACCESS TO ACTIVITY IN THE OPER-
      ANT CONDITIONING THERAPY OF PATIENTS WITH ANOREXIA NER-
      VOSA MAY BE RELATED TO:
      A. The persistent wish to be on the move which is characteristic of these
          patients
      B. The fact that the illness is more frequent in women
      C. Lack of cooperation in milieu therapy program
      D. Lack of motivation to improve
      E. Wish to eat secretly   Ref. 167 - p. 1096

55

338. A MARKED LACK OF LIBIDINAL AND GENITAL AROUSAL IS COMMON IN:
    A. Grand mal epilepsy
    B. Petit mal epilepsy
    C. Temporal lobe epilepsy
    D. Migraine
    E. Gerstmann's syndrome   Ref. 168 - p. 1099

339. JOHN ROMANO WOULD ENCOURAGE THE MEDICAL STUDENT WHO
    DECIDES TO BECOME A PSYCHIATRIST TO:
    A. Start a psychoanalysis during his first year of medical training
    B. Work concomitantly in a graduate course in one of the social sciences
    C. Take his elective training during medical school in psychiatry
    D. Obtain as broad an experience as possible in general medicine before
       entering the field
    E. Defer the internship   Ref. 169 - p. 1125

340. THE GREATEST OBSTACLE TO ORGANIZATIONAL CHANGE IN A
    MENTAL HOSPITAL IS:
    A. High degree of segmentation
    B. Community resistance to change
    C. Lack of central leadership
    D. Staff resistance
    E. All of the above   Ref. 170 - p. 1107

341. THE WISCONSIN PLAN OF UNDERGRADUATE MEDICAL EDUCATION:
    A. Increases the number of medical school years to six years
    B. Does away with the four-year liberal arts college requirement
    C. In effect begins residency training in psychiatry in the senior year of
       medical school
    D. Discourages psychiatric training until experience in general practice
       is obtained
    E. Has been abandoned   Ref. 171 - p. 1130

342. ACCORDING TO KAUFMAN THE CURRENT FOCUS ON COMMUNITY
    PSYCHIATRY IN PSYCHIATRIC EDUCATION:
    A. Has run its course
    B. Has replaced the need to know the individual in depth
    C. Is a result of the Viet Nam War
    D. Is a major advance in psychiatric training
    E. Will lead to a reintegration of psychiatry with medicine
                                               Ref. 172 - p. 1156

343. KORO IS A PSYCHOGENIC SYNDROME IN WHICH:
    A. The patient hallucinates his double
    B. Ideas of reference predominate
    C. Mutism and aboulia are features
    D. Women tend to predominate
    E. Subjective experience of penile shrinkage occurs in association
       with acute anxiety   Ref. 173 - p. 1171

344. TRANYLCYPROMINE IS A DRUG WHICH:
    A. Discharges norepinephrine extraneuronally onto receptors
    B. Increases the neuronal uptake of norepinephrine
    C. Has a facilitory effect on monoamine oxidase
    D. Does not cause hypertensive cerebrovascular reactions
    E. None of the above   Ref. 174 - p. 925

345. ACCORDING TO GROTJAHN THE TECHNIQUE WHICH IS MOST HELPFUL
FOR AN UNDERSTANDING OF THE THERAPEUTIC PROCESS IN ONE'S
PATIENTS IS:
A. Continuous supervision
B. Tape recording of sessions
C. Occasional sessions in a one-way mirror observation
D. Note taking
E. Psychological testing   Ref. 175 - p. 936

346. IN THE PSYCHIATRIC INTERVIEW, THE DECISIVE IMPACT UPON THE
DIAGNOSTIC DECISION IS MADE MOST OFTEN DURING THE FIRST:
A. Minute
B. Three minutes
C. Thirty minutes
D. Session
E. None of the above   Ref. 176 - p. 972

347. NOT CHARACTERISTIC OF THE PASSIVE-AGGRESSIVE PERSONALITY
DISORDER IS:
A. Interpersonal strife
B. Physical aggressiveness
C. Manipulative behavior
D. Outburst of anger
E. Impulsivity   Ref. 177 - p. 980

348. THE FIRST AUTHOR TO USE AND DEFINE THE TERM "MENTAL STATUS"
WAS:
A. Kraepelin
B. Eugen Bleuler
C. Adolf Meyer
D. Binet
E. Esquirol   Ref. 178 - p. 998

DIRECTIONS FOR QUESTIONS 349 - 425:

FOR EACH OF THE INCOMPLETE STATEMENTS BELOW, ONE OR MORE
OF THE COMPLETIONS IS CORRECT. SELECT:

A. If only 1, 2, and 3 are correct
B. If only 1 and 3 are correct
C. If only 2 and 4 are correct
D. If only 4 is correct
E. If all are correct

349. CINANSERIN, AN ANTISEROTONIN AGENT:
1. Produces a remission of the manic phase of manic-depressive psychosis
2. Has a mechanism of action similar to methysergide
3. Is effective in the management of symptoms associated with malignant
carcinoid syndrome
4. Is effective in the treatment of schizophrenia
          Ref. 179 - p. 1020

350. METHYSERGIDE, AN ANTISEROTONIN AGENT:
1. Is effective in the treatment of schizophrenia
2. Produces vascular insufficiency syndromes
3. Is effective in the treatment of mania only after several weeks
4. Is effective in mania within 48 hours of beginning treatment
Ref. 179 - p. 1020

351. THE SYMPTOMS OCCURRING IN NARCOLEPSY ARE:
1. Hypersomnolence
2. Cataplexy
3. Sleep paralysis
4. Hypnagogic hallucinations
Ref. 180 - p. 1027

352. WHEN SLEEP PARALYSIS OCCURS:
1. It does so during the first period of rapid eye movements
2. It does so during the stages 3 and 4 of sleep
3. There is a breakdown in the synergistic control of consciousness and motor activity
4. It is always associated with narcolepsy   Ref. 180 - p. 1028

353. MORITA IS:
1. A Japanese method of treating neurosis
2. Characterized by an initial period of absolute bed rest
3. A work-oriented therapy
4. A psychosis occurring in the Far East   Ref. 181 - p. 1032

354. THE PHENOMENON OF TOLERANCE TO THE EFFECTS OF CHLORPROMAZINE:
1. Develops to the sedative effects
2. Develops to the antipsychotic effects
3. Develops to the hypotensive effects
4. Does not occur   Ref. 182 - p. 294

355. TOTAL BODY POTASSIUM:
1. Is consistently elevated in mania
2. Is consistently elevated in depression
3. Is consistently depressed in mania and depression
4. Is not affected by lithium carbonate in therapeutic doses
Ref. 183 - p. 300

356. VARIATIONS IN TOTAL BODY WATER (TRITIUM SPACE):
1. Do not occur in manic-depressive disease
2. Accompany mood changes in manic-depressive disorders
3. Cannot be correlated with the mood changes in affective disorders
4. Appear to be stabilized by lithium in affective disorders
Ref. 184 - p. 303

357. THE PLASMA CORTISOL LEVELS WITH LITHIUM THERAPY:
1. Show an increase related to lithium alone
2. Show a decrease related to lithium alone
3. Have no relation to the phase of illness or remission
4. Show no change related to lithium alone   Ref. 185 - p. 355

358. THE PATIENT WHO LEAVES THE HOSPITAL AGAINST MEDICAL ADVICE:
1. Usually would not benefit from further treatment
2. Has been less involved in the treatment program
3. Usually has been in the hospital longer than the average patient
4. Often has alcoholism as part of his problem
Ref. 186 - p. 355

359. AS CHARACTERIZED BY GENERAL SYSTEMS THEORY, AN OPEN SYSTEM:
1. Interacts dynamically with its environment
2. Takes in elements and puts out products
3. Maintains a homeostatic steady state
4. Develops increasingly complex states of organization
Ref. 187 - p. 364

360. IN THE THERAPEUTIC MILIEU:
1. There is a reflection of current society's more egalitarian attitudes as opposed to medical-hierarchical ones
2. Lines between staff and patient groups are often not clear-cut
3. Staff problems are often discussed with patients
4. Are found the criteria of an open system
Ref. 187 - p. 360

361. DELTA SLEEP (SLOW WAVE, STAGES 3 AND 4):
1. Is promoted by exercise in animals and man
2. Is a deep sleep according to criteria involving cerebral responsiveness of ease of arousal
3. Is higher on exercise days of subjects who exercise regularly
4. Drop significantly over the month of exercise restriction in subjects who previously exercised regularly
Ref. 188 - p. 369

362. IN SUBJECTS WHO UNDERGO A ONE-MONTH DEPRIVATION OF EXERCISE PERIOD AFTER HAVING PREVIOUSLY EXERCISED REGULARLY:
1. There is an increase in REM density
2. Increase in sexual tension is reported
3. There is an increased need to be with others
4. More frequent awakenings are noted
Ref. 188 - p. 369

363. SIGNS OF IMPAIRED SLEEP ARE:
1. More frequent awakening
2. Decreased sleep depth
3. Longer sleep latencies
4. Shorter sleep latencies
Ref. 189 - p. 368

364. PHASES OF THE REACTION TO BLINDNESS ARE:
1. Disbelief
2. Protest
3. Depression
4. Recovery or continuation as a pathological syndrome
Ref. 189 - p. 379

365. THE TURNING POINT IN THE INITIAL DISTRESS REACTION TO LOSS OF SIGHT:
1. Is related to whether loss of sight was gradual or sudden
2. Is akin to the end of a period of mourning
3. Occurs in all blind persons
4. Is associated with increased self-esteem from attempting and mastering self-sufficient acts
Ref. 189 - p. 373

366. MAJOR DETERMINANTS FOR FAVORABLE ADJUSTMENT TO BLINDNESS ARE:
1. Total or near-total blindness
2. Forthright acknowledgment of the condition
3. Treatment in a high-morale center with expectations of resumption of activity
4. Partial blindness   Ref. 189 - p. 377

367. THEORIES WHICH HAVE BEEN ADVANCED TO EXPLAIN THE SYMPTOMS OF SCHIZOPHRENIA INCLUDE:
1. Sensitivity to affective stimuli
2. Social censure
3. Regression
4. Interference   Ref. 190 - p. 194

368. IN TERMS OF A SIMILARITY BETWEEN THE HUMAN MIND AND PROGRAMMABLE COMPUTERS CONSTRUCTED OF UNRELIABLE COMPONENTS, RELIABILITY OF OPERATION CAN BE IMPROVED BY:
1. Duplicating operations
2. Time pressure
3. Simultaneously running several versions of the same program
4. Novelty   Ref. 190 - p. 206

369. SCHIZOPHRENIC THOUGHT DISORDER HAS BEEN COMPARED TO THE MODEL OF A COMPUTER THAT IS:
1. Overworked
2. Underworked
3. Broken down
4. Noisy   Ref. 190 - p. 206

370. OXIDATIVE BIOTRANSFORMATION OF CHLORPROMAZINE OCCURS IN THE LIVER BY:
1. Sulphoxidation
2. Hydroxylation
3. Demethylation
4. Methylation   Ref. 191 - p. 214

371. THE METABOLISM OF CHLORPROMAZINE IS CHARACTERIZED BY:
1. A plasma level half-life of 2 - 31 hours
2. Stimulation by phenobarbital treatment
3. Peak plasma levels in two to four hours after administration, and decline to predosage levels within 12 hours
4. Urinary excretion of mainly unmetabolized parent compound
                    Ref. 191 - p. 215

372. PLASMA FREE FATTY ACID CONCENTRATION TENDS TO BE:
1. Elevated in schizophrenia
2. Elevated in depressed patients
3. Depressed in depressed patients
4. A measure of free fatty acids released by adipose tissue
                    Ref. 192 - p. 221

373. ADOLESCENT PATIENTS WITH AFFECTIVE DISORDER:
1. Are rare
2. Tend to have family histories of affective disorder, alcoholism, or both
3. Usually do not experience remission of symptoms
4. Are more likely to show severe or prolonged illness on follow-up
   if psychotic at index admission   Ref. 193 - p. 263

374. ADOLESCENTS WITH ENURESIS TEND TO HAVE PARENTS WHO:
1. Are in conflict severe enough to threaten dissolution of the home
2. Tend to be uninvolved with the handling of the enuretic problem
3. Discipline inconsistently and encourage acting out
4. Show open preference for the enuretic as opposed to the other siblings
                                        Ref. 194 - p. 244

375. PATIENTS WITH CHARACTEROLOGICAL PROBLEMS WHO ARE INSIS-
TENTLY DEMANDING AND WHO MAKE CLINGING PLEAS FOR HELP:
1. Frustrate and threaten the therapist by the urgent atmosphere they
   generate
2. May have experienced defective mothering in childhood
3. Have needs which cannot be articulated in a mature adult setting
4. Require drugs rather than psychotherapy
                                        Ref. 195 - p. 248

376. ENGEL'S FAMOUS PATIENT, MONICA:
1. Suffered from an esophageal stricture as a neonate
2. Was marasmic at five months and reacted to strangers with hypotonic
   withdrawal
3. Eventually received corrective surgery
4. Was attractive and active in adolescence, but was not autonomous
   and usually managed to get the other person to structure the situation
                                        Ref. 195 - p. 250

377. THE CHARACTEROLOGICAL PROBLEM OF MANIC-DEPRESSIVE
PATIENTS INCLUDES:
1. Envy and competition
2. Lack of ambivalence
3. Extraordinary perceptiveness to interpersonal subtleties on a level
   below consciousness
4. Strong drive for independence   Ref. 196 - p. 252

378. THE SPOUSES OF PATIENTS WITH MANIC-DEPRESSIVE PSYCHOSES:
1. Tend to be more tolerant of the illness than do spouses of patients
   with unipolar depressive illness
2. Have a significantly different attitude from that of spouses of patients
   with unipolar depressive illness
3. Rarely consider separation or divorce
4. Are often motivated to dissolve the mariage
                                        Ref. 196 - p. 258

379. IN THE TREATMENT OF THE MANIC-DEPRESSIVE PATIENT, THE
APPROACH TO DECREASE MANIC SYMPTOMATOLOGY IS:
1. Focusing on the feelings which underlie the manic's behavior
2. Open acknowledgment of conflicting feeling about the patient
3. Logically conceptualizing the manic's interpersonal activity
4. Unambivalent, firm and even arbitrary setting of limits and controls
Ref. 196 - p. 261

380. THE "PRAECOX FEELING" INDUCED IN THE OBSERVER WHICH RUMKE
CONSIDERS THE ONLY VALID DIAGNOSTIC CRITERION OF
SCHIZOPHRENIA INCLUDES:
1. A sense of uneasiness
2. A sense of distance
3. A sense of unfamiliarity
4. Difficulty in understanding   Ref. 197 - p. 266

381. STRONG FEELINGS IN THE HOSPITAL STAFF OF A "WISH TO RESCUE"
ARE ELICITED BY:
1. Manic patients
2. Depressed patients
3. Paranoid patients
4. Young acute schizophrenic patients   Ref. 197 - p. 265

382. IN TERMS OF THE EMOTIONAL RESPONSE ELICITED IN THE HOSPITAL
STAFF, THE MANIC PATIENT:
1. May be irritating and provoking anger
2. May provoke warmth and humor
3. Often has a contagious quality in his affect
4. Induces a sense of unfamiliarity   Ref. 197 - p. 265

383. THE PARANOID PSYCHOTIC MAY ELICIT FEELINGS IN THE STAFF OF:
1. Contagion
2. Fear
3. Irritation
4. Puzzlement   Ref. 197 - p. 265

384. PATIENTS WHO HAVE BEEN PREVIOUSLY DIAGNOSED AS
SCHIZOPHRENIC SHOULD BE CONSIDERED FOR A TRIAL OF LITHIUM
WHEN:
1. There are recurrent acute episodes of psychosis with delusional
thinking and hyperactivity
2. Prepsychotic personality is indicative of successful interpersonal
relationships
3. Periods between psychotic episodes are essentially symptom-free
4. Affective lability, distractibility stimuli, and engagement with others
are present during the psychotic episode
Ref. 197 - p. 262

385. GHETTO CHILDREN WERE FOUND TO BE MORE ACCESSIBLE TO
GROWTH THROUGH A PRESCHOOL EXPERIENCE WHEN THEY WERE:
1. Not divided into separate groups on the basis of IQ scores
2. Allowed to help one another
3. Encouraged to model themselves after the more competent members
of the group
4. Placed in separate groups corresponding to high, middle, and low
competence   Ref. 198 - p. 276

386.   SMALL SHARP SPIKES ARE OFTEN FOUND IN THE EEG OF:
1. Patients with affective disorders
2. Patients with schizophrenia
3. Patients with an increased incidence of abdominal surgery, medical problems, and complaints of anatomic dysfunction
4. Those with seizures and other CNS dysfunction
Ref. 199 - p. 283

387.   SMALL SHARP SPIKES:
1. Are occasional, inconspicuous single spikes on the EEG
2. Were first named by Gibbs and Gibbs
3. Occur during drowsiness and light sleep
4. Are found in those below age 21 mainly
Ref. 199 - p. 277

388.   THE EFFECT OF TETRAHYDROCANNABINOL ON VOLUNTEERS IN A NEUTRAL SETTING IS:
1. Experience of impaired cognition
2. Altered time sense
3. Dreamlike feelings
4. Considerable somatic discomfort   Ref. 200 - p. 104

389.   EFFECTS OF TETRAHYDROCANNABINOL WHICH ARE USUALLY NOT REPORTED IN LSD SUBJECTS ARE:
1. Feeling less control of one's body and feelings
2. Loss of time sense
3. Anxiety
4. Sedative effect   Ref. 200 - p. 103

390.   THE PROCESS OF POLARIZATION AND DEPOLARIZATION OF THE CELL MEMBRANE DEPENDS UPON THE GRADIENTS ACROSS THE CELL MEMBRANE OF:
1. Sodium
2. Lithium
3. Potassium
4. Acid-base balance   Ref. 201 - p. 108

391.   PATIENTS MAINTAINED ON A CONSTANT SODIUM DIET HAVE BEEN FOUND TO HAVE:
1. Sodium retention during depression
2. Decreased body sodium during depression
3. Decreased body sodium during recovery from depression
4. Sodium retention during recovery from depression
Ref. 201 - p. 110

392.   LITHIUM ADMINISTRATION CAUSES AN ACUTE:
1. Saluresis
2. Kaluresis
3. Increase in urine volume
4. Decrease in urine volume   Ref. 201 - p. 113

393. A GROUP OF YOUNG ADULT PSYCHIATRIC PATIENTS WHICH DOES NOT HAVE A SIGNIFICANTLY HIGHER INCIDENCE OF NEUROLOGIC ABNORMALITY IS:
1. Schizophrenia
2. Males as opposed to females
3. Females as opposed to males
4. Affective disorders   Ref. 202 - p. 118

394. ACCORDING TO THE CRITERIA OF HERTZIG AND BIRCH, NEUROLOGICAL ABNORMALITY IS DEFINED AS THE PRESENCE OF:
1. At least one hard sign
2. At least two hard signs
3. At least two soft signs
4. At least one hard sign and one soft sign
                                            Ref. 202 - p. 115

395. THE FOLLOWING ARE HARD SIGNS OF CNS DYSFUNCTION:
1. Lateralizing cranial nerve findings
2. Unequivocally abnormal EEG findings
3. Pathological reflexes
4. Localizing findings of CNS abnormality
                                            Ref. 202 - p. 115

396. THE FOLLOWING ARE SOFT SIGNS OF CNS DYSFUNCTION:
1. Extinction to bilateral simultaneous stimulation
2. Bilateral marked hyperreflexia
3. Score of less than 10 on the Auditory-Visual Integration Test
4. Localizing finding of CNS abnormality
                                            Ref. 202 - p. 115

397. THE MANIFEST CONTENT OF DREAMS IN NORMAL SUBJECTS GENERALLY:
1. Contains two characters in addition to the dreamer
2. Occurs out of doors
3. Is more passive than active
4. Is more pleasant than unpleasant   Ref. 203 - p. 151

398. SO-CALLED "TYPICAL DREAMS" INCLUDE DREAMS OF:
1. Being chased
2. Being naked
3. Taking an examination
4. Being rescued   Ref. 203 - p. 151

399. SEX DIFFERENCES IN MANIFEST DREAM CONTENT INCLUDE:
1. Women being more frequently the other characters in the dreams of women
2. Women having more exposure themes
3. Women expressing less ambivalence toward both sexes than do men
4. Women having more passive dreams than men
                                            Ref. 203 - p. 152

64

400. DREAMS WHICH ARE THOUGHT TO BE UNIQUE TO SCHIZOPHRENIA
HAVE A MANIFEST CONTENT OF:
1. A frightening, banal quality
2. Frightening, rapidly changing scenes
3. An isolated actionless object
4. Briefness and barren quality   Ref. 203 - p. 154

401. THE MANIFEST DREAMS OF SCHIZOPHRENICS MAY BE CHARACTER-
IZED AS:
1. Unrealistic
2. Affectively neutral
3. Openly hostile with the hostility directed at the dreamer
4. Less blatantly sexual than waking life
                                          Ref. 203 - p. 154

402. THE MANIFEST DREAM CONTENT OF THE DEPRESSED PATIENT:
1. Tends to be reported at great length with vivid detail
2. May be affectively depressed in tone
3. Shows an increase in anxiety and hostility coincident with clinical
improvement
4. Shows an increase in sexuality and mobility coincident with improvement
                                          Ref. 203 - p. 155

403. THE DREAMS OF THE MENTALLY RETARDED ARE CHARACTERIZED
BY:
1. Usually being pleasant
2. Being unrelated to day residues
3. Having themes of going home, going to parents, and going away from
the institution
4. Having a nightmare-like quality   Ref. 203 - p. 155

404. THE MANIFEST DREAMS OF THOSE WITH ORGANIC BRAIN DAMAGE
DEVELOPING LATE IN LIFE TEND TO BE:
1. Unpleasant
2. Apparently unrelated to day residues
3. Having themes of lost resources and bodily defects
4. Having themes of being small children in their parents'home
                                          Ref. 203 - p. 155

405. ACCORDING TO KENNISTON, A NEW DEVELOPMENTAL STAGE OF
LIFE CALLED "THE STAGE OF YOUTH":
1. Has emerged as a result of increasing affluence and technology of
present-day society
2. Whose crisis can be summarized as individuation versus alienation
3. Has as its task finding or creating congruence between the individual
and existing institutions
4. Occurs just prior to adolescence   Ref. 204 - p. 169

406. BLOS CHARACTERIZES LATE ADOLESCENCE AS A PERIOD OF:
1. Impoverishment and depletion
2. Integration and consolidation
3. Arrogance and rebelliousness
4. Defining goals and life tasks   Ref. 204 - p. 167

407. ERIKSON DESCRIBES THE PSYCHOSOCIAL CRISIS OF YOUNG ADULT-
HOOD AS BEING:
1. Industry vs. inferiority
2. Identity vs. identity diffusion
3. Generativity vs. self-absorption
4. Intimacy vs. isolation   Ref. 204 - p. 167

408. DRUGS USED FOR FACILITATING PSYCHIATRIC AND THERAPEUTIC
INTERVIEWS INCLUDE:
1. Barbiturates (e.g., amobarbital)
2. Steroids (e.g., hydroxydione)
3. Amphetamines (e.g., methamphetamine)
4. Folic acid analogs (e.g., methotrexate) Ref. 205 - p. 2

409. THE CLINICAL SYNDROME OF ENDOGENOUS DEPRESSION IS SEEN
MOST COMMONLY IN:
1. Outpatient clinics
2. Emergency treatment units
3. Day hospital units
4. Inpatient units   Ref. 206 - p. 21

410. GENERAL RECOMMENDATIONS FOR THE PLANNING OF RESEARCH
ON THE EFFECTIVENESS OF PSYCHOTHERAPY WOULD INCLUDE:
1. The theoretical basis for the treatment and the concept presumed to
be indexed should be indicated
2. Measurement procedures should be standardized, and measures
developed in the context of other theoretical orientations should be
included
3. Specification of details about the treatment, setting, patients, and
measuring operations to enable replication by other investigators
4. Avoidance of modes of psychotherapy based on the unconscious
                                            Ref. 207 - p. 23

411. NIGHTS WITH LONG FOURTH DREAM PERIODS HAVE BEEN FOUND
TO BE:
1. Preceded by psychotherapy sessions characterized by self-satisfied,
wish-fulfilled, controlled and elated state
2. Preceded by psychotherapy sessions characterized by depressed, less
controlled, less self-satisfied, less fulfilled and more anxious state
3. Followed by psychotherapy sessions characterized by depressed,
less controlled, less self-satisfied, less fulfilled and more anxious
state
4. Followed by psychotherapy sessions characterized by self-satisfied,
wish-fulfilled, controlled and elated state
                                            Ref. 208 - p. 38

412. HIGHER THAN NORMAL DREAM TIME HAS BEEN FOUND:
1. To have a positive correlation with anxiety
2. Following dream deprivation
3. In some borderline patients
4. In some depressions   Ref. 208 - p. 33

413.   THE ELECTROLYTE CHANGES IN PATIENTS WITH AFFECTIVE
       DISORDERS TREATED WITH LITHIUM CARBONATE ARE:
       1. An increase in 24-hour sodium space
       2. An increase in extracellular fluid volume
       3. A decrease in residual sodium
       4. A decrease in 24-hour exchangeable sodium
                                          Ref. 209 - p. 44

414.   CHILDREN WHO SET FIRES:
       1. Are usually boys
       2. Tend to manifest a sense of exclusion, loneliness   and unfulfilled
          dependency needs
       3. Attempt to gratify infantile masturbatory impulses
       4. Are usually well into adolescence   Ref. 210 - p. 71

415.   LITHIUM CARBONATE:
       1. Was introduced into psychiatry by Cade, of Australia, in 1949
       2. Should not exceed a serum concentration of 0.6 mEq/liter
       3. Is prepared in 300 mg capsules which contain 8.12 mEq of lithium
          per capsule
       4. Is contraindicated when the patient is depressed
                                          Ref. 211 - p. 73

416.   THE SYMPTOMS SEEN IN THE CONCENTRATION CAMP SYNDROME
       INCLUDE:
       1. Episodic depression
       2. Anxiety state
       3. Obsessive rumination over the past
       4. Feeling of emptiness, despair, and hopelessness
                                          Ref. 212 - p. 86

417.   THE TRANSFERENCE NEUROSIS:
       1. Is a nosological term
       2. Can develop in a patient with schizophrenia
       3. Is identical to the concept of transference
       4. Is an operational concept which refers to events in analysis
                                          Ref. 213 - p. 22

418.   THE TRANSFERENCE NEUROSES:
       1. Are characterized by a patient's suggestibility and capacity to form a
          transference
       2. Are contrasted to narcissistic neuroses
       3. Are a nosological group
       4. Include the psychoses   Ref. 213 - p. 22

419.   TRANSFERENCE IS:
       1. Limited to therapeutic relationships
       2. Usually conscious
       3. Does not occur in children
       4. A displacement of aspects of an unconscious mental representation
          of an infantile object into a mental representation of a current external
          object   Ref. 214 - p. 42

420. IN PSYCHOANALYSIS, THE ESSENSE OF THE THERAPY IS:
1. Development of the transference neurosis
2. Analysis of the transference neurosis
3. Resolution of the transference neurosis
4. Maintenance of the transference neurosis
Ref. 215 - p. 83

421. THE TERM "AMENTIA" HAS BEEN USED FOR:
1. Dementia
2. Mental retardation
3. Certain confusional states
4. Schizophrenia   Ref. 216 - p. 779

422. THE TERM "KORSAKOW'S PSYCHOSIS" HAS BEEN USED TO DESCRIBE:
1. Alcoholic hallucinations
2. Alcoholic dementia combined with polyneuritis
3. Pathological intoxication
4. Amnestic-confabulatory syndrome regardless of etiology
Ref. 216 - p. 779

423. THE TERM "NEUROSIS" WHEN ORIGINALLY INTRODUCED REFERRED
TO:
1. Unconscious conflict
2. Psychogenic symptoms not psychotic in quality
3. Psychopathy
4. Disorders caused by organic brain damage
Ref. 216 - p. 785

424. THE TERM "PSYCHOSIS" WHEN ORIGINALLY INTRODUCED REFERRED
TO:
1. The break with reality
2. The entire personality being affected by the disorder
3. Disturbed and disordered behavior
4. Mental symptoms caused by organic brain damage
Ref. 216 - p. 785

425. REACTIVE PSYCHOSES WHICH APPEAR IN THE EIGHTH EDITION OF
THE INTERNATIONAL CLASSIFICATION OF DISEASE, BUT ARE
BRACKETED (AND THEREFORE TO BE AVOIDED IN THE UNITED STATES)
BY DSM-II INCLUDE:
1. Reactive excitation
2. Reactive confusion
3. Acute paranoid reaction
4. Psychotic depressive reaction   Ref. 216 - p. 785

68

DIRECTIONS FOR QUESTIONS 426 - 432:

MATCH EACH AUTHOR WITH THE TERM HE INTRODUCED:

A. Galen
B. Von Feuchtersleben
C. Cullen
D. Bleuler
E. Kasanin

426. ___ Neurosis
427. ___ Psychosis
428. ___ Schizoaffective psychosis
429. ___ Ambivalence
430. ___ Autism
431. ___ Amentia
432. ___ Dereistic thinking   Ref. 216 - pp. 779, 782, 783, 785

FOR EACH OF THE FOLLOWING INCOMPLETE STATEMENTS, CHOOSE
THE COMPLETION THAT IS MOST APPROPRIATE:

433. ADAPTIVE PSYCHOTHERAPY IS A TERM APPLIED TO THE PSYCHO-
THERAPEUTIC TECHNIC THAT AIMS AT THE FOLLOWING, EXCEPT:
A. Fostering the adjustment of the patient
B. Addressing itself to the patient's specific disabling problem
C. Addressing itself to the patient's maladaptation
D. Springing from ego-syntonic and adaptive derivatives within the
therapist
E. Fostering the adaptation of the patient
Ref. 217 - p. 792

434. ADAPTIVE PSYCHOTHERAPY IS CHARACTERIZED BY THE FOLLOWING,
EXCEPT:
A. Patient contact over an extended, often indefinite period of time
B. Contacts generally less frequent than weekly, but lasting a full
50 minutes
C. Frequent use of drugs
D. Technics which include support, institutional alliance, advice, and
environmental manipulation
E. Being specifically designed for the chronically ill psychotic patient
Ref. 217 - p. 792

435. ADAPTATION IS DIFFERENTIATED FROM ADJUSTMENT IN THAT:
A. Adjustment is regressive
B. Adaptation is progressive
C. Adjustment implies passive submission to societal goals
D. Adaptation is not tolerated by society
E. Adjustment implies intrapsychic arrest
Ref. 217 - p. 792

436. THE ADMINISTRATION OF PSYCHOTROPIC DRUGS ON A ONE DOSE
PER DAY SCHEDULE IS POSSIBLE BECAUSE:
A. These drugs have a long biological half-life
B. Their metabolism and excretion proceed at a low rate
C. Tissues release accumulations of these drugs very slowly
D. Antipsychotic and antidepressant effects are noted later in time than
are secondary properties
E. All of the above   Ref. 218 - p. 796

437. INTERMITTENT DRUG THERAPY:
   A. Has been found to be ineffective in the treatment of schizophrenia
   B. Can be utilized when excretion of metabolites is rapid
   C. Involves drug-free weekends
   D. Induces a feeling of dependence on the drug in the patient
   E. Causes greater accumulation of the drug in body organs
   Ref. 218 - p. 800

438. THE REPORT OF THE NATIONAL ADVISORY COMMISSION ON CIVIL DISORDER IMPLICATED AS THE MAJOR CAUSE OF BLACK AND WHITE CONFLICT AND VIOLENT CIVIL DISORDERS:
   A. Absence of the father or significant male figure in the home
   B. Dissolution of the family
   C. Poverty amidst affluence
   D. City life and its effect on poor minorities
   E. White racism
   Ref. 219 - p. 802

439. FORMS OF RACISM INCLUDE:
   A. Extremism
   B. Moderate
   C. Reform
   D. Occasional manifestations of racist response resulting from growing up in a racist society
   E. All of the above
   Ref. 219 - p. 805

440. THE PSYCHOLOGICAL ROOTS OF RACISM ARE:
   A. Will to power
   B. Projection of unacceptable unconscious impulses
   C. Self-awareness
   D. Group pride
   E. Genetic
   Ref. 219 - p. 804

441. COMPARISON OF THE ACCIDENT RATES OF INDIVIDUALS OPERATING MOTOR VEHICLES REVEALS THAT:
   A. Schizophrenics have a higher rate than controls
   B. Schizophrenics have a lower rate than controls
   C. Controls have a higher rate than personality and psychoneurotic disorders
   D. Personality disorders and psychoneurotic disorders have a higher rate than controls
   E. Schizophrenics have a higher rate than personality and psychoneurotic disorders
   Ref. 220 - p. 807

442. SCHIZOPHRENICS WHO OPERATE MOTOR VEHICLES:
   A. Have a rate of violations for drunken driving similar to the general population
   B. Have a rate of violation for reckless driving similar to the general population
   C. Have a rate of violation for negligent driving similar to the general population
   D. Have a rate of violation for defective equipment similar to the general population
   E. Have a rate of violation for improper turns similar to the general population
   Ref. 220 - p. 811

70

443. KLINEFELTER'S SYNDROME CONSISTS OF THE FOLLOWING, EXCEPT:
   A. Gynecomastia
   B. Aspermia
   C. Hypogonadism
   D. Feminine fat distribution
   E. Short stature   Ref. 221 - p. 814

444. KLINEFELTER'S SYNDROME HAS A CHROMOSOME KARYOTYPE OF:
   A. XO
   B. XY
   C. XXY
   D. XYY
   E. XXYY   Ref. 221 - p. 814

445. THE MOST FREQUENT PSYCHOLOGICAL MANIFESTATION OF THE
   KLINEFELTER SYNDROME IS SOME FORM OF PERSONALITY DISORDER
   WHICH IS TYPICALLY:
   A. Antisocial
   B. Passive-dependent
   C. Inadequate-schizoid
   D. All of the above
   E. None of the above   Ref. 221 - p. 815

446. IN KLINEFELTER'S SYNDROME:
   A. Mental retardation is usually mild when it does exist
   B. Barr bodies are present in the buccal smear
   C. A majority of the individuals marry
   D. All of the above
   E. None of the above   Ref. 221 - p. 815

447. T-GROUPS:
   A. Were first developed by Moreno as an adjunct to his psychodrama
   B. Are task-oriented groups
   C. Are designed to strengthen poor ego defenses
   D. Are long-term, ongoing groups
   E. Grew out of a project to train community leaders to deal with inter-
      racial problems   Ref. 222 - p. 824

448. IN THE LABORATORY GROUP METHOD DEVELOPED AT BETHEL,
   MAINE:
   A. A-groups were developed to analyze immediate interaction
   B. T-groups focused on structural group task exercises
   C. A-groups rapidly metamorphosed into T-groups unless strenuous
      efforts were made to keep the A-groups task-oriented
   D. All of the above
   E. None of the above   Ref. 222 - p. 825

449. LIABILITIES OF THE T-GROUP METHOD INCLUDE:
   A. Lack of adequate participant-selection criteria
   B. Lack of clearly defined responsibility
   C. Fostering a concept that anything goes, regardless of consequences
   D. All of the above
   E. None of the above   Ref. 222 - p. 834

450. UNDER T-GROUPS ARE SUBSUMED:
   A. Sensitivity, personal encounter groups
   B. Task-oriented groups involving structured group exercises aimed at teaching group function skills
   C. Intervention laboratories that are established for functional work groups in the community or industry
   D. All of the above
   E. None of the above   Ref. 22 - p. 827

451. THE T-GROUP IS CHARACTERIZED BY:
   A. Aiming to increase self-awareness and "authenticity" of life experiences
   B. The leader becoming fully assimilated in the group
   C. Elaboration, analysis and discussion of conscious thought and feeling interpersonal interaction, and "here and now" issues
   D. All of the above
   E. None of the above   Ref. 222 - p. 827

452. PEOPLE WHO COULD BE INCLUDED IN T-GROUPS ARE:
   A. Psychotic individuals
   B. Characterologic neurotics
   C. Hysterics
   D. Individuals in crisis
   E. None of the above   Ref. 223 - p. 842

453. KURT LEWIN IS ASSOCIATED WITH THE DEVELOPMENT OF:
   A. Esalen
   B. Phoenix House
   C. National Training Laboratory
   D. Daytop Village
   E. Marathons   Ref. 223 - p. 840

454. THE HUMAN RELATIONS TRAINING LABORATORY:
   A. Is a four-week program
   B. Utilizes Development Groups or D-Groups
   C. Is designed to deal with patients rather than non-patients
   D. Is self-governed and participants create their own rules
   E. All of the above   Ref. 224 - p. 858

455. THE LEADER OF A SENSITIVITY TRAINING GROUP:
   A. Is required by law to remain responsible once he has undertaken a professional relationship
   B. Must maintain records
   C. Must remain available to the members of the group unless he formally discontinues his responsibility in writing
   D. All of the above
   E. None of the above   Ref. 255 - p. 871

456. LEADERS OF T-GROUPS:
   A. Are required to obtain the consent of the individuals involved in the group
   B. Are scientifically or medically qualified persons
   C. Minimize the degree of risk to the individuals involved in the group
   D. All of the above
   E. None of the above   Ref. 255 - p. 871

72

457. THE REVISED STANDARDS FOR PSYCHIATRIC FACILITIES, PUBLISHED
IN 1969 BY THE AMERICAN PSYCHIATRIC ASSOCIATION:
A. Require that a qualified psychiatrist be the head of any psychiatric
facility
B. Covers psychiatric facilities for children
C. Defines standards of patient-personnel ratios
D. All of the above
E. None of the above   Ref. 226 - p. 880

DIRECTIONS FOR QUESTIONS 458 - 467:

MATCH EACH PERSON WITH THE CONCEPT WITH WHICH HE IS
ASSOCIATED:

A. C.G. Carus
B. J.E. Purkinje
C. Lord Chief Justice Tindal
D. Justice Charles Doe
E. E. von Hartmann

458. ___ M'Naghten rule
459. ___ New Hampshire rule
460. ___ Anticipated concept of the unconscious, dichotomy of introvert vs.
extrovert, and correlation of morphological types and mental illness
461. ___ Described three levels of the unconscious
462. ___ Value of dreams for the study of the personality
                                        Ref. 227 - pp. 894,893,892

MATCH EACH PERSON WITH THE CONCEPT WITH WHICH HE IS
ASSOCIATED:

A. Morgagni
B. Francis Galton
C. George Miller Beard
D. Harvey Cushing
E. William Healy

463. ___ Child guidance movement
464. ___ Opposed notion of a homogeneous treatment for mental disease by
showing there is no uniform cerebral pathology for mental disorder
465. ___ Concept of hyper- versus hypo-pituitarism
466. ___ Used free associations to demonstrate significance of childhood
memories upon adulthood
467. ___ 19th Century American civilization conducive to neurasthenia
                                        Ref. 227 - pp. 896,892,895

73

FOR EACH OF THE FOLLOWING INCOMPLETE STATEMENTS, CHOOSE
THE COMPLETION THAT IS MOST APPROPRIATE:

468. THE SOCIAL SECURITY LAW PROVIDES THAT IN ORDER TO QUALIFY
FOR DISABILITY BENEFITS:
   A. An applicant must be unable to engage in gainful activity
   B. An applicant must have a physical or mental impairment which can
      be expected to result in death
   C. An applicant has to have had his impairment for a continuous period
      of not less than 12 months
   D. All of the above
   E. None of the above   Ref. 228 - p. 898

469. IN THE SOCIAL SECURITY ADMINISTRATION DISABILITY DETERMI-
NATIONS:
   A. Signs carry more weight than symptoms
   B. The psychiatric consultant must submit conclusions with his findings
   C. The mental status examination is not a source for factual evidence
   D. A battery of psychological tests is required
   E. The psychiatric consultant is the one who makes the final determination
      of disability   Ref. 228 - p. 898

MATCH EACH PERCENTAGE OF CONCORDANCE FOR SCHIZOPHRENIA
IN MONOZYGOTIC TWINS WITH THE APPROPRIATE STUDY:

   A. 80%
   B. 30%
   C. 15%
   D. 2%
   E. None of the above

470. ___ National Academy of Sciences-National Research Council study of
         15,909 veteran twin pairs
471. ___ Kallman's study
472. ___ Kringlen's Norway study using national cohorts rather than hospital
         referrals
473. ___ Tienari's Finland study using national cohorts rather than hospital
         referrals
474. ___ Burlingham's study of twins   Ref. 229 p. 604

SELECT THE MOST APPROPRIATE COMPLETION IN THE FOLLOWING
MULTIPLE CHOICE QUESTIONS:

475. IN THE NAS-NRC STUDY OF 15,909 PAIRS OF VETERAN TWINS THE
PRESENCE OF A GENETIC FACTOR:
   A. Is not suggested for the pathogenesis of schizophrenia
   B. Appears to be present in the pathogenesis of schizophrenia
   C. Is suggested by the higher concordance rate for schizophrenia in
      dizygotic twins
   D. Is of significance in the pathogenesis of schizophrenia since 85% of
      monozygotic twins were concordant
                                   Ref. 229 - p. 597

74

476. THE MONOZYGOTIC/DIZYGOTIC CONCORDANCE RATIO FOR
SCHIZOPHRENIA IN THE NAS/NRC STUDY:
A. Is no higher than the rate seen in psychoneurosis
B. Is of the same order as that for fractures
C. Is of the order of 3.3:1
D. Suggests that heredity is the major factor in the pathogenesis of
schizophrenia
E. Approaches that seen in Kallman's classic study
Ref. 229 - p. 597

477. THE METHODOLOGICAL PROBLEMS INHERENT IN TWIN STUDIES FOR
THE DETERMINATION OF THE ROLE OF HEREDITY IN MENTAL
DISORDERS INCLUDE:
A. The nature of the sample
B. Zygosity determination
C. Differences attendant on incomplete or incorrect diagnosis
D. All of the above
E. None of the above
Ref. 229 - p. 610

478. THE GROUP OF 15,909 PAIRS OF SAME-SEXED VETERAN TWINS MAY
BE BIASED BECAUSE OF THE PROBABLE EXCLUSION OF:
A. Reactive schizophrenics
B. Process schizophrenics
C. Affective disorders
D. Character disorders
E. Psychoneuroses
Ref. 229 - p. 610

479. THE HIGHEST PERCENTAGE OF CHROMOSOME BREAKAGE OCCURS
WHEN HUMAN LEUKOCYTES ARE CULTURED WITH:
A. LSD-25
B. Ergonovine maleate
C. Aspirin
D. Streptonigrin
E. Phytohemagglutinin
Ref. 230 - p. 633

480. CHROMOSOME BREAKAGE IN HEAVY USERS OF LSD:
A. Has not been found to be higher than in controls in recent studies
B. Is often lower than that seen with controls
C. Is lower than the amount seen in subjects on phenothiazines
D. Occurs in significant amounts when these users are young children
with schizophrenia who received the drug experimentally
E. Has not been found in any study
Ref. 230 - p. 626

481. PARENTS OF CHILDREN WITH SEVERE PHYSICAL DISEASE USUALLY:
A. Blame the doctor
B. Exhibit inappropriate guilt
C. Withdraw from the child
D. Visit faith healers
E. Require psychotherapy
Ref. 231 - p. 636

482. BEGINNING IN APRIL 1969, THE NATIONAL ASSOCIATION OF BLUE
SHIELD PLANS:
   A. Discontinued coverage of outpatients' treatment in psychiatry
   B. Requires that outpatient psychiatric treatment be available as a paid
   in full benefit to insured groups willing to buy it
   C. Covers outpatient psychiatric treatment and reimburses 50% of the
   total cost
   D. Offers outpatient psychiatric treatment coverage of the deterrent type
   E. Has a limit of $500 per year for outpatient psychiatric treatment
   Ref. 232 - p. 671

483. THE FIRST YEAR OF THE UNITED AUTO WORKERS PSYCHIATRIC
BENEFIT PROGRAM WAS CHARACTERIZED BY THE FOLLOWING,
EXCEPT:
   A. Laying of stress on outpatient care
   B. Being economically viable
   C. Utilization rate of 6.4 per 1,000 eligible persons
   D. Decrease in in-hospital utilization
   E. Average number of visits was 8.5   Ref. 233 - p. 675

484. THE PSYCHIATRIC SERVICES IN THE SOUTHERN CALIFORNIA PER-
MANENTE MEDICAL GROUP IS CHARACTERIZED BY THE FOLLOWING,
EXCEPT:
   A. Outpatient psychiatric services
   B. Majority of patients are in classes IV and V
   C. Were found to be overutilized in the area of outpatient psychotherapy
   D. Coverage of union employees
   E. Coverage of federal employees
   Ref. 234 - p. 681

485. SEXUAL ACTIVITY IS THOSE OVER 60:
   A. Is rare
   B. Declines more sharply than the rate of decline in previous decades
   C. Continues when there is proper health and proper environment
   D. Declines more sharply for women than for men
   E. Occurs but with diminished satisfaction
   Ref. 235 - p. 713

486. THE ILLEGAL DRUG ALMOST ALWAYS FIRST USED BY RUNAWAYS IS:
   A. Heroin
   B. Methedrine
   C. STP
   D. Marijuana
   E. Barbiturates   Ref. 236 - p. 719

487. RUNAWAYS AND HIPPIES TEND TO CONSIDER AS A DESIRABLE
EFFECT OF THE ABOVE DRUG:
   A. Apathy
   B. Depression
   C. Diminished aggressiveness
   D. Loss of motivation
   E. Diminished energy   Ref. 236 - p. 719

488. AN IMIPRAMINE ANTIDEPRESSANT REGIMEN IS ENHANCED BY THE
ADDITION OF:
A. Reserpine
B. Tetrabenazine
C. MAO inhibitors
D. All of the above
E. None of the above   Ref. 236 - p. 719

489. A GROUP OF PATIENTS WHO APPEAR TO BE RELATIVELY REFRAC-
TORY TO IMIPRAMINE INCLUDES:
A. Hyperthyroid depressed patients
B. Hypothyroid depressed patients
C. Schizophrenic depressed patients
D. Aged depressed patients
E. Involutional depressed patients   Ref. 237 - p. 463

490. WHEN SMALL DOSES OF TRIIODOTHYRONINE ARE COMBINED WITH
USUAL DOSES OF IMIPRAMINE:
A. A more rapid improvement in retarded depressed patients is produced
B. Toxicity is increased
C. There is a slight but definite shift toward hyperthyroidism
D. Ankle reflexes become slowed
E. Manic reactions are more frequently reported
          Ref. 237 - p. 466

491. THE ADDITION OF T3 TO IMIPRAMINE:
A. Is more effective for agitated depressions than retarded depressions
B. Leads to an increased incidence of cardiovascular side effects
C. Has greater effectiveness in the aged
D. Has greater effectiveness in men
E. Has greater effectiveness in women   Ref. 237 - p. 464

492. THE CONCEPT THAT DEPRESSION IS ASSOCIATED WITH A DEFICIENCY
OF NOREPINEPHRINE AT FUNCTIONALLY IMPORTANT ADRENERGIC
RECEPTOR SITES IN THE BRAIN IS A STATEMENT OF THE:
A. Catecholamine hypothesis
B. Indolealkylamine hypothesis
C. Adenyl cyclase hypothesis
D. Thyroid hypothesis
E. Electrolyte hypothesis   Ref. 237 - p. 457

493. IN BOTH HUMANS AND MICE IMIPRAMINE IS MORE TOXIC IN THE
PRESENCE OF:
A. Adrenogenic syndrome
B. Addison's disease
C. Severe hyperthyroidism
D. Severe hypothyroidism
E. Severe anemia   Ref. 237 - p. 458

494. THE RELATIVE RISK OF DEATH FOR A PSYCHIATRIC CARE GROUP
COMPARED TO THE GENERAL POPULATION IS:
A. The same
B. 2.5:1
C. 1:1 when the chronically ill, aged, and alcoholic are removed
D. 1:1.5
E. None of the above   Ref. 238 - p. 478

495. THE HIGHEST RATE OF IMPROVEMENT IN ALCOHOLIC PATIENTS OCCURS WITH:
A. LSD with therapist present
B. LSD without therapist present
C. Amobarbital and methedrine given with therapist present
D. Routine clinic care
E. None of the above   Ref. 239 - p. 486

496. DEATH RESULTING FROM THE EFFECTS OF PROLONGED SLEEPLESS-NESS HAS BEEN REPORTED IN:
A. Laboratory experiments involving prolonged sleep deprivation
B. Temporal lobe epilepsy
C. Bell's mania
D. Military personnel stationed in the South Pole
E. Imipramine toxicity   Ref. 240 - p. 495

497. AFTER PROLONGED SLEEP DEPRIVATION ALL OF THE FOLLOWING ARE NOTED, EXCEPT:
A. Increased plasma 17-OHCS levels
B. Disruption of circadian pattern
C. Decrease in Stage IV and REM sleep in the recovery period
D. Nystagmus   Ref. 240 - p. 496

498. FOLLOWING 205 HOURS OF SLEEP DEPRIVATION, SUBJECTS WERE FOUND TO BE:
A. Flattened in effect
B. Impaired in their functioning for several weeks
C. Depressed
D. Paranoid
E. Evidencing no delayed psychological sequellae
          Ref. 240 - p. 495

499. VARIABLES WHICH ARE HIGHLY CORRELATED WITH REMISSION IN SCHIZOPHRENIA INCLUDE THE FOLLOWING, EXCEPT:
A. Confusion
B. Gradual onset
C. Concern with death
D. Depressive heredity
E. Non-schizoid premorbid adjustment   Ref. 241 - p. 500

500. FACTORS WHICH ARE HIGHLY CORRELATED WITH A PROCESS SCHIZOPHRENIC CLASSIFICATION INCLUDE THE FOLLOWING, EXCEPT:
A. Schizoid personality
B. Manic-depressive features
C. Insidious onset
D. Inadequate heterosexual relationships
E. Reality distortion   Ref. 241 - p. 400

501. TRICHOTILLOMANIA:
A. Is more common in boys
B. Does not occur before age 2
C. Is not found after age 10
D. Is found in the elated phase of affective disorders
E. Is more frequent in girls   Ref. 242 - p. 505

502. THE FORENSIC PSYCHIATRIST:
A. Must hold membership in the American Academy of Forensic Psychiatry
B. Must have a practical working knowledge of the law
C. Currently has a clear role and identity
D. All of the above
E. None of the above   Ref. 243 - p. 525

503. THE FORENSIC PSYCHIATRIST REQUIRES COMPETENCE IN:
A. Pre-trial evaluation
B. Post-trial treatment
C. Training and research
D. All of the above
E. None of the above   Ref. 243 - p. 519

504. THE CNS OF LSD INCLUDE THE FOLLOWING, EXCEPT:
A. Low voltage fast pattern on the EEG
B. Irregular slowing on the EEG
C. Seizure activity in the EEG recorded from limbic region of cats
D. Paroxysmal activity in the hippocampal and septal regions
of schizophrenics with chronically implanted electrodes
E. Paroxysmal activity in the amygdala of schizophrenics with chronically
implanted electrodes   Ref. 244 - p. 537

505. THERE IS A PRINCIPLE IN LAW WHICH STATES THAT TEMPORARY
INSANITY BROUGHT ON BY VOLUNTARY INTOXICATION:
A. Is no defense for criminal behavior
B. Is a legitimate defense for criminal behavior
C. Is no defense with alcohol, but is a defense with narcotics, barbiturates,
tranquilizers, and other mind-altering chemicals
D. Is a defense for felonies, but not for misdemeanors
E. Is a defense only in the State of New York
                                        Ref. 244 - p. 536

506. SUFFICIENT GROUNDS FOR A DETERMINATION OF LEGAL INSANITY
MAY BE:
A. Delirium
B. Organic psychosis
C. Delirium tremens
D. All of the above
E. None of the above   Ref. 244 - p. 536

507. LSD EXPERIENCES ARE ASSOCIATED WITH THE FOLLOWING, EXCEPT:
A. Improved concentration
B. Time and space distortion
C. Mood swings
D. Frequent paranoid feelings
E. Hallucinations almost invariable concomitant
                                        Ref. 244 - p. 536

508. IN THE TASK THAT CONFRONTS THE PSYCHIATRIST EXAMINING AN INDIVIDUAL WHO HAS BEEN ACCUSED OF COMMITTING A CRIME WHILE UNDER THE INFLUENCE OF A HALLUCINOGENIC DRUG AND WHO PLEADS NOT GUILTY BY REASON OF INSANITY:
   A. It is necessary to establish that the crime did occur during the period in which the person was psychotic
   B. It is necessary to establish that the psychotic state was of such magnitude as to significantly influence the commission of the crime
   C. It is necessary to establish whether a drug-induced psychosis existed
   D. One must convince a jury that the accused's mental state at the time the crime was committed meets the requirements of the legal test of insanity
   E. All of the above   Ref. 244 - p. 534

509. IN ENGLAND A RELATIVE MAY PETITION COMPULSORY HOSPITAL ADMISSION FOR:
   A. An emergency
   B. Observation
   C. Treatment
   D. All of the above
   E. None of the above   Ref. 245 - p. 538

510. THE MENTAL HEALTH INFORMATION SERVICE OF NEW YORK STATE:
   A. Was established in 1965
   B. Has a staff based at the state hospitals
   C. Has a staff which informs patients of their legal rights
   D. Has a staff which provides the court with relevant information about the patient's case
   E. All of the above   Ref. 245 - p. 541

511. THE 1967 DELIBERATIONS OF THE PRESIDENT'S COMMISSION ON LAW AND JUSTICE RECOMMENDS:
   A. Training law enforcement and court officers to be more sensitive to signs of mental abnormality
   B. Abandonment of commitment procedures
   C. Use of non-medical diagnostic services
   D. All of the above
   E. None of the above   Ref. 246 - p. 548

512. HALLUCINATORY SEIZURES:
   A. May represent any of the sensory modalities
   B. Involve a "doubling of consciousness"
   C. May reproduce "strips of memory"
   D. Are symptomatic of a discharging focus in the temporal lobe
   E. All of the above   Ref. 247 - p. 561

513. PERCEPTUAL ILLUSIONS:
   A. Include "deja vu" phenomena
   B. Are false interpretations of real sensory stimuli
   C. Include micropsia, macropsia, and distortions of hearing
   D. As psychical seizures involve pathology in the nondominant temporal lobe
   E. All of the above   Ref. 247 - p. 562

514. MOOD OR EMOTIONAL CHANGES AS PSYCHICAL SEIZURES INCLUDE TRANSITORY:
   A. Feelings of fear
   B. Feelings of well-being
   C. Depressive feelings lasting several minutes to 14 days
   D. Feelings of terror followed by a hallucination of smell or taste
   E. All of the above   Ref. 247 - p. 563

515. IN THE FORCED THINKING OF PSYCHICAL SEIZURES:
   A. The patient can usually remember the exact thought or thoughts
   B. The patient describes recurring and compelling thoughts which enter his mind and all other thoughts are excluded
   C. The psychodynamic basis is similar to obsessional thinking
   D. The pathology is rarely in the frontal lobes
   E. All of the above   Ref. 247 - p. 563

516. PSYCHICAL SEIZURES:
   A. May be followed by a generalized seizure
   B. Usually are not associated with a disturbance of consciousness
   C. Are not associated with automatisms
   D. Are often neurotic in their pathogenesis
   E. All of the above   Ref. 247 - p. 561

517. FLASHBACKS:
   A. Are recurrent intrusions into awareness long after the ingested hallucinogenic drug has worn off
   B. Are most common in the auditory modality
   C. Are usually not frightening to the subject
   D. Do not occur following use of marijuana
   E. May be associated with severe anxiety but do not constitute a psychiatric emergency   Ref. 248 - p. 567

518. REPORTS OF SUDDEN DEATH FROM ASPHYXIATION ON FOOD:
   A. Have been attributed to the use of tranquilizers
   B. Started to appear following the introduction of reserpine and chlorpromazine in clinical use
   C. May be due to frequent abnormalities in the swallowing mechanism in schizophrenic patients
   D. All of the above
   E. None of the above   Ref. 249 - p. 572

519. THE USE OF MONOZYGOTIC TWINS FOR RESEARCH INTO PERSONALITY FORMATION PROVIDES THE FOLLOWING ADVANTAGE:
   A. Genetic determinants of personality differences between twins are not identical
   B. Other variables, including socioeconomic class, ethnic background, and age differ
   C. Comparisons of physical and psychological development can be made with one twin serving as a control
   D. Intrafamilial relationships do not differ
   E. Birth experiences are similar   Ref. 250 - p. 1597

81

520. IN THE STUDY OF INFANT TWINS, MOTHER LINKAGE (CLEAR-CUT PREFERENCE OR GREATER INVOLVEMENT) IS ASSOCIATED AT BIRTH WITH:
A. The second born
B. The smaller
C. The neurologically inferior
D. All of the above
E. None of the above
Ref. 250 - p. 1600

521. FATHER LINKAGE IS ASSOCIATED WITH THE TWIN WHO AT BIRTH:
A. Is the first born
B. Has the lower Apgar score
C. Is neurologically inferior
D. Is smaller
E. Is weaker
Ref. 250 - p. 1600

522. WITHIN THE MONOZYGOTIC TWIN RELATIONSHIP ONE TWIN IS FREQUENTLY:
A. More dominant
B. Larger
C. More active-curious
D. All of the above
E. None of the above
Ref. 250 - p. 1601

523. AT THE AGE OF ONE YEAR, DEPENDENCE IN A TWIN IS ASSOCIATED WITH:
A. High Apgar score
B. Mother linkage
C. Father linkage
D. The first born
E. The less curious-active
Ref. 250 - p. 1601

524. ESSENTIAL FOR THE VALID ASSESSMENT OF THE EFFICACY OF ANTIDEPRESSANT DRUGS IS:
A. The inclusion of a group receiving ECT
B. The inclusion of a phenothiazine
C. The inclusion of a MAO inhibitor
D. The inclusion of a tricyclic antidepressant
E. The inclusion of a placebo
Ref. 251 - p. 1605

525. A DRUG WHICH IS INFERIOR TO PLACEBO IN THE ANTIDEPRESSANT SCALE IS:
A. Nortriptyline
B. Amitriptyline
C. Diphenylhydantion (Dilantin)
D. Amitriptyline-diazepam
E. Amitriptyline-perphenazine
Ref. 251 - p. 1609

526. METHYLPHENIDATE POTENTIATES THE ACTION OF:
A. Phenothiazines
B. Reserpine
C. Barbiturates
D. Imipramine
E. Alcohol
Ref. 252 - p. 1619

527. RITALIN TREATMENT OVER A 14 DAY PERIOD INHIBITS THE METABOLISM OF:
   A. Thorazine
   B. Stelazine
   C. Tofranil
   D. All of the above
   E. None of the above   Ref. 252 - p. 1624

528. THE RESPONSE OF A DEPRESSION TO IMIPRAMINE WOULD BE IMPROVED BY THE ADDITION OF:
   A. Diphenylhydantoin (Dilantin)
   B. Coumarin
   C. Methylphenidate
   D. Insulin
   E. Vitamin B_{12} Ref. 252 - p. 1624

529. FOLLOW-UP STUDIES SHOW THAT HOSPITAL READMISSION RATES CAN BE LOWERED BY:
   A. Hospital stays longer than one month but shorter than six months
   B. Hospital stays longer than six months but shorter than one year
   C. Intensive psychotherapy during the inpatient stay
   D. Milieu therapy
   E. Follow-up care   Ref. 253 - p. 1630

530. THE BODY BUFFER ZONE IS HIGHER IN MAGNITUDE IN:
   A. Aggressive prisoners
   B. Nonaggressive prisoners
   C. Nonschizophrenics as opposed to schizophrenics
   D. Hysterics
   E. Obsessionals   Ref. 254 - p. 1644

531. THE AREA OF GREATEST SENSITIVITY TO APPROACH OF THE BODY BUFFER ZONE IS:
   A. The rear
   B. The front
   C. The eyes
   D. The mouth
   E. The head   Ref. 254 - p. 1644

532. BASED ON THE PREDRINKING BEHAVIOR IT IS:
   A. Impossible to predict how an alcoholic will act when drinking begins
   B. Usually possible to predict how an alcoholic will act when drinking begins
   C. Usually possible to recognize in the behavior of an alcoholic when he is drinking, an exaggeration of the predrinking behavior
   D. Usually possible to estimate the limit of alcohol that the alcoholic can tolerate
   E. Possible to predict which alcoholic will experience delirium tremens
                                           Ref. 255 - p. 1651

533. THE RESULTS OF PSYCHOTHERAPY WITH CHRONIC ALCOHOLICS:
   A. Are good if the patients are well motivated
   B. Are better in women than in men
   C. Are better in those who avoid wine
   D. Are improved by the use of phenothiazines
   E. Are unsatisfactory   Ref. 255 - p. 1650

534. THE ALCOHOLIC "BLACKOUT" IS:
A. An amnesia for significant events that occurred during a drinking episode
B. Rarely of concern to the alcoholic
C. Due to malingering
D. All of the above
E. None of the above   Ref. 256 - p. 1659

535. MARKED IMPAIRMENT OF SHORT-TERM MEMORY FUNCTION OCCURS IN:
A. Temporal lobe epilepsy
B. Transient global amnesia
C. Following bilateral temporal lobe surgery
D. Blackouts in chronic alcoholics   Ref. 256 - p. 1663

536. THE MECHANISM OF THE SHORT-TERM MEMORY IMPAIRMENT IN ALCOHOLIC BLACKOUTS INVOLVES:
A. Registration
B. Retention
C. Recall
D. All of the above
E. None of the above   Ref. 256 - p. 1664

537. ANOTHER TYPE OF "BLACKOUT" OCCURRING IN ALCOHOLICS, IN WHICH THERE IS REALIZATION OF THE FORGOTTEN EVENT WHEN IT IS RECALLED SPONTANEOUSLY OR BROUGHT TO THE PERSON'S ATTENTION, IS MORE LIKELY CAUSED BY A DEFECT OF:
A. Registration
B. Retention
C. Recall
D. All of the above
E. None of the above   Ref. 257 - p. 1665

538. THE ANTEROGRADE AMNESIA OBSERVED IN ALCOHOLIC "BLACKOUTS" PROBABLY INVOLVES:
A. The frontal lobes
B. Globus pallidus
C. Corpus striatum
D. Hippocampus
E. Thalamus   Ref. 257 - p. 1669

539. ACTIVATION OF SEXUAL BEHAVIOR IS FOUND FOLLOWING THE USE OF:
A. Lithium carbonate
B. L-dopa
C. Thioridazine
D. Haloperidol
E. Heroin   Ref. 258 - p. 1691

540. STIMULUS INTENSITY CONTROL:
A. Refers to the manner in which an individual automatically modulates sensory stimulation
B. Was originally inferred from performances on a kinesthetic size-judgment task
C. Divides subjects into two groups: augmenters and reducers
D. All of the above
E. None of the above   Ref. 259 - p. 501

84

541. AUGMENTATION OF THE AVERAGE EVOKED RESPONSE ON THE EEG
TO INCREASES OF THE INTENSITY OF THE VISUAL STIMULUS OCCURS:
A. In bipolar disorder patients
B. In unipolar affective disorder patients
C. With lithium carbonate administration in both bipolar and unipolar
patients
D. All of the above
E. None of the above   Ref. 259 - p. 503

542. REDUCTION OF AVERAGE EVOKED RESPONSE AMPLITUDE WITH
INCREASING INTENSITY OF THE VISUAL STIMULUS OCCURS:
A. With lithium carbonate administration in unipolar patients
B. With lithium carbonate administration in bipolar patients
C. In unipolar patients
D. All of the above
E. None of the above   Ref. 259 - p. 503

543. THE COMBINATION OF TRICYCLIC ANTIDEPRESSANTS AND MONOAMINE
OXIDASE INHIBITORS:
A. Has been avoided in the United States and Great Britain
B. Leads to morbidity in a high percentage of patients
C. Is not more effective than one or the other drug given alone
D. All of the above
E. None of the above   Ref. 260 - p. 509

544. IN THE COMBINED THERAPY OF TRICYCLIC ANTIDEPRESSANT AND
MAOI:
A. Imipramine is preferred to amitriptyline
B. Treatment should be initiated with both drugs simultaneously
C. Treatment should be begun with the MAOI and the tricyclic should
be added subsequently
D. Treatment should be begun with the tricyclic and the MAOI should be
added subsequently
E. Phenothiazines should be avoided   Ref. 260 - p. 513

545. WHEN TRICYCLICS AND MAOI ARE USED IN COMBINED TREATMENT:
A. Foods high in tyramine content should be strictly avoided
B. Over the counter cold medications may be used cautiously
C. Amphetamines may be used in small amounts
D. Barbiturates are contraindicated
E. Phenothiazines are contraindicated   Ref. 260 - p. 513

546. THE BEHAVIORAL PARADIGM WHICH CLARIFIES THE PARADOXICAL
DEPRESSION THAT SOMETIMES OCCURS AFTER "SUCCESS" IS:
A. Loss of reinforcers
B. Loss of operants
C. Negative reinforcement
D. Positive reinforcement
E. Operant conditioning   Ref. 261 - p. 522

547. MONOAMINE OXIDASE IS HIGHER IN THE BRAIN, PLASMA, AND
PLATELETS OF:
A. Younger compared to older subjects
B. Women compared to men
C. Whites compared to blacks
D. All of the above
E. None of the above   Ref. 262 - p. 536

548.   THE DIFFERENCES IN LEVELS OF MONOAMINE OXIDASE ARE COMPAT-
        IBLE WITH THE CLINICAL FINDINGS THAT:
        A.   Mania is more common in men than in women in the older age groups
        B.   Depression is more frequent in women
        C.   Major depressive illnesses occur more frequently with advancing age
        D.   All of the above
        E.   None of the above   Ref. 262 - p. 539

549.   DREAM RECALL TENDS TO BE FAVORED BY:
        A.   Abrupt awakening
        B.   Early in the night REM period awakenings
        C.   Presleep tension
        D.   Fatigue
        E.   Awakening during stage 4   Ref. 263 - p. 550

550.   THE EEG EFFECT OF DIPHENHYDRAMINE (BENADRYL) IN CHILDREN
        IS:
        A.   Generalized increase in fast waves
        B.   Fast alpha waves
        C.   High voltage 4 to 6 cycle per second activity
        D.   All of the above
        E.   None of the above   Ref. 264 - p. 552

551.   THE EEG EFFECT OF THORAZINE IN CHILDREN IS:
        A.   Slow alpha
        B.   Generalized slowing
        C.   Well correlated with clinical behavioral changes
        D.   All of the above
        E.   None of the above   Ref. 264 - p. 562

552.   THE TEMPORAL DISTORTION INDUCED BY MARIJUANA CONSISTS OF:
        A.   Changes in the sense of duration
        B.   Confusion in the past, present and future
        C.   Changes in temporal perspective
        D.   All of the above
        E.   None of the above   Ref. 265 - p. 564

553.   INCREASED CONCENTRATION ON THE PRESENT, ALONG WITH REMOTE-
        NESS OF THE PAST AND FUTURE, ARE FEATURES OF ALTERED CONS-
        CIOUSNESS WHICH OCCUR:
        A.   During hypnotic and meditative states
        B.   During intoxication with mescaline and LSD
        C.   During intoxication with marijuana
        D.   All of the above
        E.   None of the above   Ref. 265 - p. 566

554.   INCREASED LEVELS OF CREATINE PHOSPHOKINASE AND ALDOLASE
        ARE PRESENT IN THE SERUM OF A SIGNIFICANT PERCENTAGE OF
        ACUTELY PSYCHOTIC PATIENTS:
        A.   If their symptomatology is in the affective sphere
        B.   Provided they are studied during the initial weeks of psychotic
             decompensation
        C.   Only when the diet is high in tyramine-containing foods
        D.   In the presence of phenothiazines
        E.   When they are carriers of the Duchenne-type pseudohypertrophic
             muscular dystrophy   Ref. 266 - p. 568

555. THE MANAGEMENT AND TREATMENT OF PSYCHIATRIC CASUALTIES
      IN WAR ZONES IS BASED ON THE PRINCIPLE OF:
      A. Immediacy
      B. Proximity
      C. Expectancy
      D. All of the above
      E. None of the above   Ref. 267 - p. 289

556. TO MANAGE PSYCHIATRIC CASUALTIES IN THE VIET NAM COMBAT
      ZONE IN 1967-1968 THE ARMY UTILIZED:
      A. 100 psychiatrists
      B.   50 psychiatrists
      C.   20 psychiatrists
      D.   5 psychiatrists
      E.   2 psychiatrists   Ref. 267 - p. 289

557. BRIEF PSYCHOTIC EPISODES USUALLY WITH PREDOMINANTLY PARA-
      NOID SYMPTOMATOLOGY ARE A SYNDROME THAT PHYSICIANS IN VIET
      NAM HAVE COME TO ASSOCIATE WITH:
      A. Combat fatigue
      B. Marijuana usage
      C. Bitter feelings in the combat troops related to resentment of
          those in the peace movement in the United States
      D. Confusion over the basis of the war
      E. Inability to identify the enemy   Ref. 267 - p. 295

558. AN IMPORTANT MODALITY OF THE TREATMENT WARD IN THE
      VIET NAM WAR ZONE IS:
      A. Psychoanalysis
      B. Exploratory psychotherapy
      C. Milieu therapy
      D. Insulin coma treatment
      E. Hypnotherapy   Ref. 267 - p. 297

559. THE INTENSIVE TREATMENT MILIEU WHICH IS EFFECTIVE IN
      LIMITING REGRESSION IN SCHIZOPHRENIC PATIENTS:
      A. Is inappropriate for the treatment of depression
      B. Has a low staff-patient ratio
      C. Does not provide for psychotherapy
      D. Is not integrated with the community
      E. May induce a massive behavioral disturbance in some patients with
          character or borderline disturbances
                                         Ref. 268 - p. 300

560. METHODS OF COPING WITH BEHAVIORAL REGRESSIONS IN THE IN-
      TENSIVE TREATMENT MILIEU WHEN PSYCHOTHERAPY, MEDICATIONS
      RESTRICTIONS, AND SPECIAL ATTANDANTS PROVED INEFFECTIVE
      INCLUDE:
      A. Insulin coma treatment
      B. Hydrotherapy
      C. Family therapy
      D. Therapeutic transfer to a large state hospital
      E. Community involvement   Ref. 268 - p. 300

561. THE BEHAVIORAL DISTURBANCE OF BORDERLINE PATIENTS IN THE INTENSIVE TREATMENT MILIEU INCLUDE:
A. Mutism, self-inflicted lacerations, window breakage, and verbal and physical abuse of the staff
B. Encouraging other disturbed patients to use narcotics, escape from the hospital, or make suicide attempts
C. Manifest "envy" of sicker patients and the techniques of management required by severely regressed or suicidal patients such as special nurses or EST
D. Actions that are more destructive of the milieu than similar acts by schizophrenic patients
E. All of the above   Ref. 268 - p. 300

562. ASPECTS OF THE PSYCHOPATHOLOGY OF THE BORDERLINE PATIENTS WITH THE ABOVE BEHAVIORAL DISTURBANCES INCLUDE:
A. Primitive and magical beliefs about other people
B. Sense of entitlement that justifies actions toward frustrating individuals
C. Need for immediate gratification
D. Use of the defense of projection
E. All of the above   Ref. 268 - p. 302

563. PRINCIPLES OF SUCCESSFUL INPATIENT TREATMENT OF THE ABOVE PATIENTS INCLUDE:
A. Stirring up the patient so that he may understand his inner conflicts
B. Providing the patient with the possibility of "working through"
C. Hospitalization of three to six months in duration
D. Use of drugs
E. Avoidance of therapy that is aimed at providing the patient with a "good relationship"   Ref. 268 - p. 302

564. THE "NEW CHRONIC PATIENTS IN MENTAL HOSPITALS REPLACING SCHIZOPHRENICS" ARE:
A. Borderline patients with behavioral disturbances
B. Affective disorders
C. LSD-induced psychoses
D. Alcoholics
E. Viet Nam War veterans who are drug addicts
          Ref. 268 - p. 304

565. THE IN-HOSPITAL TREATMENT OF BORDERLINE PATIENTS WITH BEHAVIORAL DISTURBANCES SHOULD:
A. Not focus on the transference relationship except to clarify the therapist's limited role in the patient's life
B. Find immediate goals for the hospitalization
C. Be limited to three months, although an even shorter period is desirable
D. Enlist the entire therapeutic community to set strict limits on the disruptive behavior
E. All of the above   Ref. 268 - p. 302

88

566. HIGH DOSES OF TRIFLUOPERAZINE IN CHRONIC SCHIZOPHRENIA:
A. Are most effective in long-term patients
B. Are most effective in short-term patients who had been on a piperadine phenothiazine prior to the use of this drug
C. Are not effective in those patients who had previously been on an aliphatic phenothiazine
D. Are most effective in patients who were for a short term in the hospital and who had previously been on a piperazine phenothiazine
E. None of the above   Ref. 269 - p. 305

567. PEOPLE WHO CALL A SUICIDE PREVENTION CENTER:
A. Tend to be men
B. Usually do not present a suicide risk
C. Call for a friend in the majority of cases
D. Usually have an acute interpersonal crisis
E. Have a depressed mood as the motive for calling
                                              Ref. 270 - p. 314

568. OF THE 10,920 MURDERS IN THE UNITED STATES IN 1966, A CHILD WAS KILLED BY ITS OWN PARENT IN ONE OUT OF:
A. 16
B. 22
C. 40
D. 75
E. 92   Ref. 271 - p. 325

569. ASIDE FROM THOSE CASES OF FILICIDE WHICH ARE APPARENTLY ACCIDENTAL, THE APPARENT MOTIVE IS:
A. Altruistic
B. Psychotic
C. Unwanted child
D. Spouse revenge
E. All of the above   Ref. 271 - p. 325

570. THE INCIDENCE OF FILICIDE IS HIGHER IN:
A. Fathers
B. Mothers
C. Parents over 35
D. Nonpsychotic disorders
E. Cases in which the child is eight years and older
                                              Ref. 271 - p. 327

571. THE PSYCHIATRIST AS AN AMICUS CURIAE:
A. Is directly responsible to the judge
B. Makes availible his opinion and reports to the prosecution
C. Makes availible his opinion and reports to the defense
D. All of the above
E. None of the above   Ref. 272 - p. 342

572. A PHENOMENON WHICH CAN BE OBSERVED TO SOME DEGREE IN ALL PATIENTS FOLLOWING OPEN HEART SURGERY IS:
A. Euphoria
B. Catastrophic reaction
C. Transient delirium
D. All of the above
E. None of the above   Ref. 273 - p. 353

573. THE HIGHEST MORTALITY FOLLOWING OPEN HEART SURGERY IS
FOUND IN THE GROUP OF PATIENTS WHO PREOPERATIVELY WERE:
   A. Depressed
   B. Symbiotic
   C. Anxious
   D. Adjusted
   E. Denying   Ref. 273 - p. 348

574. THE INCREASED INCIDENCE OF DELIRIUM IN PATIENTS WHO UNDERGO
OPEN HEART SURGERY IS DEPENDENT UPON:
   A. The time on the cardiopulmonary bypass
   B. The environment of the open heart recovery room
   C. The role of postoperative incapacitation
   D. All of the above
   E. None of the above   Ref. 274 - p. 360

575. FOLLOWING OPEN HEART SURGERY A POOR PROGNOSIS IS ASSOCIATED
WITH THOSE PATIENTS WHO PREOPERATIVELY HAD:
   A. Schizophrenia
   B. Organic brain syndrome
   C. Psychoneurotic disorders
   D. Personality trait disturbances
   E. Personality pattern disturbances   Ref. 274 - p. 367

576. IN PATIENTS WITH PREOPERATIVE PSYCHIATRIC PROBLEMS THERE
IS A GREATER RISK FOLLOWING OPEN HEART SURGERY OF:
   A. Mortality
   B. Delirium
   C. Euphoria
   D. Depression
   E. Reoperation   Ref. 274 - p. 367

577. THE FACTORS WHICH MAY INFLUENCE THE DEVELOPMENT OF A
DELIRIUM IN CARDIOTOMY PATIENTS INCLUDE THE FOLLOWING,
EXCEPT:
   A. Increased permeability of the blood-brain barrier
   B. Reconstitution of catecholamine metabolism in heart and lung tissue
   C. Improvement of circulating normal or abnormal biogenic amines
   D. Influence of circulating normal or abnormal biogenic amines
   E. Use of high doses of intravenous antibiotics
                                         Ref. 274 - p. 368

578. THE EARLIEST SIGN IN THE DEVELOPMENT OF A DELIRIUM IS:
   A. Lability of affect
   B. Impairment of judgment
   C. Decreased vigilance and awareness as reflected in impairment of
      serial subtraction
   D. Disorientation
   E. Hallucination   Ref. 274 - p. 367

579. IN THE RESOLUTION OF THE POST-SURGERY DELIRIUM IN CARDIOTOMY
PATIENTS:
A. Orientation for person returns before orientation for time
B. Orientation for time returns before orientation for person
C. Orientation for place returns before orientation for person
D. Orientation for time returns before orientation for place
E. Orientation for person returns after orientation for time
Ref. 274 - p. 368

580. IN THE SYMPTOMATOLOGY OF ORGANIC BRAIN SYNDROME OF ACUTE
ONSET:
A. Visual hallucinations precede auditory hallucinations
B. Disorientation for place precedes disorientation for time
C. Resolution of the delirium involves the disappearence of symptoms
and signs in the order of their appearance
D. Impairment of recall precedes decreased levels of awareness
E. Delusions of reference and persecution precede social misidentifications
Ref. 274 - p. 367

581. POSTOPERATIVELY THE MOST SERIOUS PSYCHIATRIC COMPLICATION
OF HEART TRANSPLANTATION HAS BEEN:
A. Delirium
B. Suicide
C. Psychosis
D. Depression
E. Anxiety state
Ref. 275 - p. 371

582. A MAJORITY OF PATIENTS WHO DIED FOLLOWING RENAL TRANS-
PLANTATION:
A. Have experienced abandonment by their families or an important figure
B. Experienced panic about the outcome of the operation to a degree not
observed among patients who survived
C. Experienced pessimism about the outcome of the operation to a degree
not observed among patients who survived
D. All of the above
E. None of the above
Ref. 276 - p. 381

583. IN OPEN HEART SURGERY PREOPERATIVE DEPRESSION IS ASSOCIATED
WITH:
A. Septicemia
B. High mortality risk
C. No significant improvement in preoperative clinical cardiac status
D. All of the above
E. None of the above
Ref. 276 - p. 386

584. THE OUTCOME OF OPEN HEART SURGERY CORRELATES WELL WITH
THE FOLLOWING, EXCEPT:
A. Previous success in coping with life stress
B. Handling of anxiety regarding surgery
C. Academic and financial success
D. Presence or absence of depression
E. The strengths of object relations
Ref. 276 - p. 386

585. THE PSYCHOTHERAPY OF THE PATIENT WHO REQUIRES PSYCHIATRIC PREPARATION FOR KIDNEY TRANSPLANT SURGERY:
    A. May be supplemented by appropriate forms of behavior therapy
    B. Should focus on significant events of the patient's early years
    C. Can be facilitated by intravenous methedrine
    D. Must aim at minimizing any feelings of dependence on the psychiatrist
    E. Should focus on the formations of a relationship with the psychiatrist who can follow him postoperatively
                                        Ref. 276 - p. 387

586. WHEN THE PREOPERATIVE PSYCHIATRIC HISTORY OF A POTENTIAL RENAL TRANSPLANT PATIENT REVEALS A SENSE OF ABANDONMENT AND ANXIETY:
    A. It may be lifesaving to postpone kidney transplantation
    B. Active psychotherapy should be instituted immediately following surgery
    C. Combined treatment with imipramine and phenelzine may prove to be highly effective
    D. Hemodialysis should be changed to peritoneal dialysis
    E. The frequency of dialysis should be increased
                                        Ref. 276 - p. 387

587. THE INCIDENCE OF POSTOPERATIVE DELIRIUM IS HIGHER IN:
    A. Females
    B. Younger patients
    C. Patients who manifest little or no preoperative anxiety
    D. Patients who use alcohol sparingly
    E. None of the above   Ref. 277 - p. 388

588. FACTORS WHICH PREDISPOSE TO AN INCREASED INCIDENCE OF POSTOPERATIVE DELIRIUM INCLUDE:
    A. The influence of age
    B. The sex of the patient
    C. Sleep deprivation in the recovery room
    D. Perceptual distortions in the recovery room
    E. All of the above   Ref. 277 - p. 388

589. THE PATIENTS WHO HAD THE BEST PROGNOSIS AFTER HEART SURGERY:
    A. Were mainly women
    B. Did not have a history of denial of illness
    C. Showed an overwhelming desire to get well
    D. Came mainly from class IV and V
    E. Verbalized freely their fears of anesthesia and surgical complication
                                        Ref. 277 - p. 393

590. POSTOPERATIVE DELIRIUM DEVELOPS MORE FREQUENTLY IN THOSE PATIENTS WHO:
    A. Undergo elective surgery rather than emergency surgery
    B. Have not previously experienced postoperative psychosis
    C. Have no family history of psychosis
    D. Belong to the upper socioeconomic class
    E. Have a history of alcoholism   Ref. 277 - p. 393

591.   EPILEPSY OF THE NONDOMINANT TEMPORAL LOBE IS ASSOCIATED
       WITH:
       A. Manic-depressive psychotic reactions
       B. Hysteria and hysterical psychosis
       C. Schizophrenic-like psychotic reactions
       D. Hallucinatory psychoses
       E. Paranoid psychoses   Ref. 278 - p. 403

592.   EPILEPSY OF THE DOMINANT TEMPORAL LOBE IS ASSOCIATED WITH:
       A. Mania
       B. Depression
       C. Hysteria
       D. Schizophrenic-like psychotic reactions
       E. All of the above   Ref. 278 - p. 403

593.   THE EMERGENCE OF PSYCHOSIS:
       A. Is inversely correlated with the incidence of generalized seizures
       B. Is inversely correlated with the severity of generalized seizures
       C. Is inversely correlated with the presence and frequency of psychomotor-
           psychosensory seizures
       D. All of the above
       E. None of the above   Ref. 278 - p. 402

594.   ANTICONVULSANT MEDICATION FREQUENTLY INDUCES:
       A. Increased frequency of seizures which resolve when medication is
           withdrawn
       B. Psychotic episodes which resolve when medication is withdrawn and
           the patient is enabled to experience seizures
       C. Structural cerebral damage
       D. All of the above
       E. None of the above   Ref. 278 - p. 402

595.   THE NEUROPHYSIOLOGICAL SYSTEM ACTIVATED BY TEMPORAL
       SEIZURES:
       A. Appears to be "antischizophrenic"
       B. Leads to periodicity
       C. Leads to chronicity
       D. Underlies neurotic phenomena
       E. Appears to be "anti-manic-depressive"
                                                  Ref. 278 - p. 403

596.   THE NEUROPHYSIOLOGICAL SYSTEM ACTIVATED DURING GENERALIZED
       SEIZURES:
       A. Appears to be "antischizophrenic"
       B. Appears to be "anti-manic-depressive"
       C. Protects against neurosis
       D. Causes minimal brain damage
       E. Leads to chronicity   Ref. 278 - p. 403

597.   LONGITUDINAL STUDY OF ABUSED CHILDREN REVEALS:
       A. No significant increase in psychopathology
       B. A high potential for becoming violent members of society when grown up
       C. That they rarely abuse their own children in later years
       D. Reaction formation to be their major defensive pattern
       E. Decreased incidence of enuresis   Ref. 279 - p. 407

598. ABUSED CHILDREN IN LATER YEARS:
A. Identify with the victim
B. Identify with the aggressor
C. Establish a pattern of inviting harm and playing the victim
D. Become the abusive parents
E. All of the above   Ref. 279 - p. 407

599. GREATER RATES OF INCREASE OF AER (AVERAGE EVOKED RESPONSE) WITH INCREASE IN STIMULUS INTENSITY ARE SHOWN BY:
A. Bipolar affective disorder patients
B. Unipolar affective disorder patients
C. Patients treated with lithium for bipolar disorder
D. Patients treated with lithium for unipolar disorder
E. Patients who have not experienced manic episodes
                                        Ref. 280 - p. 19

600. AMPLITUDE OF AER:
A. Increases with increased perception of stimulus intensity
B. Shows wide individual variation in increase related to increasing stimulus intensity
C. May decrease in some individuals with increasing intensities of photic stimulation
D. All of the above
E. None of the above   Ref. 280 - p. 19

601. SUBJECTS WHO SHOW AUGMENTATION OF THEIR AER (AVERAGE EVOKED RESPONSE) SLOPE:
A. Tend to be chronically negative in their life attitudes
B. Have low scores for depression on their MMPI
C. Have high scores in thrill- and adventure- seeking on a stimulus-seeking questionnaire
D. Are found in the category of unipolar depressed patients
E. Respond poorly to lithium   Ref. 280 - p. 24

602. AVERAGE EVOKED RESPONSE (AER) APPEARS TO BE A REFLECTION OF:
A. Inherited tendency toward development of affective disorder
B. A mechanism in the CNS that modulates the intensity of incoming signals
C. Individual intelligence
D. Mental health and adaptation
E. Response to tranquilizers and antidepressants
                                        Ref. 280 - p. 19

603. PATIENTS WITH CUSHING'S SYNDROME, ADDISON'S DISEASE, AND RECEIVING EXOGENOUS CORTICOIDS FREQUENTLY DEVELOP:
A. Schizophrenia
B. Depression and euphoria
C. Hysteria
D. Organic mental syndrome
E. Addictive tendencies   Ref. 281 - p. 31

604. THE PRODUCTION RATE OF CORTISOL IS:
A. Increased during depression
B. Increased during recovery from depression
C. Decreased during depression and decreased further following recovery
D. Unchanged during depression and increased following recovery
E. Increased by dexamethasone   Ref. 281 - p. 31

605. THE PLASMA LEVEL OF CORTISOL IS INCREASED:
A. By the administration of methopyrapone
B. By the administration of dexamethasone
C. In the evening phase of the circadian rhythm
D. In recovered compared to depressed patients
E. In controls compared to depressed patients
                                    Ref. 281 - p. 34

606. THE NARCOTIC ADDICT REHABILITATION ACT (NARA) ENACTED BY
     CONGRESS IN 1966 PROVIDES:
A. For commitment for treatment rather than prosecution for the federal
   criminal charge if the addict so chooses
B. A sentencing procedure to commit for treatment those addicts who
   have been convicted of a federal offense
C. Civil commitment for addicts who have not been charged with any
   federal offense
D. Grants to public and nonprofit private agencies to develop treatment
   programs for addicts
E. All of the above   Ref. 282 - p. 41

607. IN THE NARA AFTERCARE PROGRAM THE PERCENTAGE OF PATIENTS
     WHO USED MORPHINE-LIKE DRUGS SIX MONTHS FOLLOWING
     DISCHARGE WAS:
A. 10-20
B. 20-40
C. 40-60
D. 60-80
E. 80-90   Ref. 282 - p. 44

608. THE STUDY OF 1,881 PATIENTS DISCHARGED FROM LEXINGTON TO
     NEW YORK CITY REPORTED THAT THE PERCENTAGE WHICH BECAME
     READDICTED IN SIX MONTHS FOLLOWING DISCHARGE WAS:
A. 10-20
B. 20-40
C. 40-60
D. 60-80
E. 80-90   Ref. 282 - p. 44

609. THE PERCENTAGE OF ADDICTS REMAINING IN GOOD STANDING IN
     THE CALIFORNIA CIVIL COMMITMENT PROGRAM AS OUTPATIENTS FOR
     THREE YEARS WAS:
A. 10-20
B. 20-40
C. 40-60
D. 60-80
E. 80-90   Ref. 282 - p. 45

610. THE LEADING CAUSE OF DEATH AMONG CHILDREN IS:
A. Cancer in its various forms
B. Cardiovascular disease
C. Congenital malformations
D. Accidents
E. Infectious disease   Ref. 283 - p. 52

611. A FREQUENT FINDING IN THE LIFE HISTORY OF THE BURNED CHILD
AND HIS FAMILY IS:
   A. Parental indifference toward the burned child prior to the injury
   B. High incidence of child-beating on the part of the parents
   C. Early parental loss suffered by the parents of the burned child
   D. High incidence of psychosis in the burned children
   E. Overt psychosis in one of the parents
                                        Ref. 283 - p. 53

612. A MAJOR POSITIVE FACTOR FOR SURVIVAL IN THE BURNED CHILD IS:
   A. Absence of a sense of guilt on the part of the parents
   B. Absence of a sense of guilt on the part of the child if other siblings
      have died in the fire
   C. Hope on the part of parents and/or staff
   D. Absence of hypertension in the burned child
   E. Absence of ulcers in the burned child
                                        Ref. 283 - p. 56

613. DURING THE FIRST YEAR OF PSYCHIATRIC RESIDENCY TRAINING:
   A. Definite changes in the personality of the resident occur
   B. Various studies have found that there is an increase in depression
      occurring in the resident
   C. Residents usually decide whether their approach to patients will be
      organic or psychotherapeutic
   D. Most of the learning in the training program takes place
   E. Residents experience transient paranoid episodes
                                        Ref. 284 - p. 81

614. A FREQUENT SIDE EFFECT OF TRICYCLIC ANTIDEPRESSANT MEDI-
CATION PARTICULARLY IN PATIENTS OVER 40 YEARS OF AGE IS:
   A. Retrolental fibroplasia
   B. Phocomelia
   C. Confusional reactions
   D. Intensification of depression
   E. Grand mal seizures   Ref. 285 - p. 95

615. AN EXAMPLE OF A DRUG WITH A LOW THERAPEUTIC INDEX (RATIO
OF THE MEDIAN TOXIC DOSE TO THE MEDIAN EFFECTIVE DOSE) IS:
   A. Lithium
   B. Thorazine
   C. Mellaril
   D. Taractan
   E. Haldol   Ref. 286 - p. 100

616. INCREASE IN DIETARY SODIUM INTAKE DURING LITHIUM CARBONATE
TREATMENT IS ASSOCIATED WITH:
   A. Increase in lithium side effects
   B. Increase in manic effect and behavior
   C. Increase in serum lithium levels
   D. All of the above
   E. None of the above   Ref. 286 - p. 103

617. A DEFENDANT WOULD BE FOUND INCOMPETENT TO STAND TRIAL IF HE WAS INCAPABLE TO ADEQUATELY DEFEND HIMSELF AGAINST HIS ACCUSERS IN A COURT OF LAW BY REASON OF:
  A. Inability to understand the nature of the legal process
  B. Inability to recognize the consequences that could follow from the accusation
  C. Inability to assist legal counsel in his own defense
  D. All of the above
  E. None of the above   Ref. 287 - p. 105

618. A DEFENDANT WOULD BE FOUND INCOMPETENT TO STAND TRIAL IF HIS DIAGNOSIS IS:
  A. Schizophrenia
  B. Chronic brain syndrome
  C. Toxic psychosis
  D. All of the above
  E. None of the above   Ref. 287 - p. 108

619. A FREQUENT PRODROMAL SYMPTOM OF DELIRIUM IS:
  A. Slurred speech
  B. Psychomotor retardation
  C. Unusual restlessness
  D. Systematized delusions
  E. Disorientation   Ref. 288 - p. 112

620. A DELIRIOUS PATIENT WHO IS DISORIENTED AS TO PERSON:
  A. Displays a loss of personal identity
  B. Misidentifies those about him
  C. Will usually be oriented as to time and place
  D. All of the above
  E. None of the above   Ref. 288 - p. 115

621. THE USE OF TWIN DATA AS EVIDENCE FOR A GENETIC FACTOR IN AFFECTIVE ILLNESS DEPENDS ON THE ASSUMPTION THAT:
  A. Being a twin does not itself make one more liable to affective disorder
  B. The increased similarity between members of an MZ twin pair (as opposed to a DZ pair) is due to genetic rather than other factors
  C. The methodological problems inherent in twin data do not significantly distort the concordance rates
  D. All of the above
  E. None of the above   Ref. 289 - p. 1

622. $h^2 = \dfrac{r_{MZ} - r_{DZ}}{1 - P_\infty}$ IS A FORMULA DEVISED BY JENSEN FOR THE DETERMINATION OF:
  A. Zygosity
  B. Heritability
  C. Concordance
  D. Heterozygosity
  E. Environmental effect   Ref. 289 - p. 4

623. DISORDERS AMONG FIRST DEGREE RELATIVES OF PATIENTS WITH
AFFECTIVE ILLNESS, WHICH ARE FOUND WITH A HIGHER LIFETIME
PREVALENCE THAN IN THE GENERAL POPULATION, INCLUDE THE
FOLLOWING, EXCEPT:
A. Involutional melancholia
B. Involutional paranoid psychosis
C. Alcoholism
D. Antisocial personality
E. Neurotic depressive reaction   Ref. 289 - p. 4

624. UNIPOLAR AFFECTIVE ILLNESS IS SIMILAR TO BIPOLAR ILLNESS IN:
A. Median age of onset
B. Mortality due to suicide
C. Occurrence of episodes of hypomania while being treated for depression
with tricyclic antidepressants or with levodopa
D. Evoked cortical potentials
E. Urinary 17-hydroxycorticosteroid excretion
Ref. 289 - p. 8

625. THE MODE OF INHERITANCE WHICH IS INCONSISTENT WITH MUCH
OF THE DATA REGARDING AFFECTIVE ILLNESS IS THE HYPOTHESIS
OF:
A. Single recessive gene
B. Single dominant gene with variable penetrance
C. Polygenic mode of inheritance
D. All of the above
E. None of the above   Ref. 289 - p. 9

626. ENCOUNTER GROUP "CASUALTIES" (INDIVIDUALS WHO BECOME MORE
DISTRESSED OR WHO EMPLOY MALADAPTIVE DEFENCES FOLLOWING
ENCOUNTER GROUP EXPERIENCES) ARE MOST FREQUENT:
A. In tape groups
B. In Synanon
C. With leaders who are confrontive, intrusive and challenging while
at the same time demonstrating positive caring
D. In unstructured groups with leaders who take a laissez-faire approach
E. With authoritarian leaders   Ref. 290 - p. 22

627. ENCOUNTER GROUP CASUALTIES OCCUR WITH GREATER FREQUENCY
IN INDIVIDUALS:
A. With low self-esteem who experience rejection in the group
B. Who remain uninvolved during the encounter group experience
C. Who drop out early in the encounter experience
D. From minority groups
E. Who are religious   Ref. 290 - p. 23

628. THE EFFECT OF SOCIAL CLASS AS A MEDIATOR VARIABLE IN
NEUROTIC SYMPTOMATOLOGY IS MANIFESTED IN LOWER SOCIO-
ECONOMIC STATUS PATIENTS BY:
A. Lower levels of anxiety
B. Lower levels of depression
C. Higher levels of somatization
D. All of the above
E. None of the above   Ref. 291 - p. 36

629. IRASCIBILITY IS MANIFESTED IN SIGNIFICANTLY HIGHER LEVELS IN
PATIENTS WHO ARE:
A. White
B. Negro
C. From high socioeconomic class
D. From the middle socioeconomic class
E. None of the above   Ref. 291 - p. 38

630. CHARACTERISTICS OF MANY PSYCHIATRIC UNITS, INCLUDING SHORT-
TERM RECEIVING WARDS, CURRENTLY INCLUDE:
A. An open door policy
B. A permissive approach to the patient
C. A degree of patient government
D. A team approach to decisions
E. All of the above   Ref. 292 - p. 42

631. PATIENT GOVERNMENT WORKS BEST:
A. In psychiatric units for the treatment of acute disorders
B. In general hospitals which have psychiatric wards
C. In a facility which treats mainly patients with endogenous illness
which renders the patients socially disabled
D. In long-term therapeutic communities for patients with problems of
social deviancy
E. All of the above   Ref. 292 - p. 45

632. DEVICES NECESSITATED AT TIMES BY OPEN DOORS IN PSYCHIATRIC
UNITS INCLUDE THE FOLLOWING, EXCEPT:
A. One to one nursing supervision
B. Over-use of the seclusion room
C. Opening and closing the door as patients and staff become concerned
or relaxed
D. Patients used as door watchers
E. Camisoles   Ref. 292 - p. 43

633. OPEN DOORS IN PSYCHIATRIC HOSPITALS HAVE LED TO A MARKED
DECREASE IN:
A. Repeated elopements
B. Suicides
C. Use of psychotropic medication
D. All of the above
E. None of the above   Ref. 292 - p. 43

634. IN CERTAIN PSYCHIATRIC HOSPITALS ENTHUSIASM FOR PATIENT
GOVERNMENT HAS LED TO THE DEMOCRATIC PROCESS BEING
APPLIED TO:
A. Prescribing medication
B. Group psychotherapy
C. Decisions regarding the use of ECT
D. All of the above
E. None of the above   Ref. 292 - p. 44

635.   THE OPEN PANEL SYSTEM IS:
       A. Characteristic of the therapeutic community
       B. One variety of prepaid health insurance
       C. A replacement for a closed-door policy
       D. A method of computor diagnosis
       E. Designed for patients who have been hospitalized for long periods
           in state institutions   Ref. 293 - p. 51

636.   WHILE THE TOTAL COST OF HEALTH SERVICES FOR THE UNITED
       STATES IS $_____ ; THE GOVERNMENT SPENDS $_____ FOR
       MENTAL HEALTH SERVICES PER YEAR:
       A. 100 million; 10 million
       B. 1 billion; 500 million
       C. 50 billion; 5 billion
       D. 50 billion; 25 billion
       E. 100 billion; 50 billion   Ref. 293 - p. 53

637.   BECK INVENTORY SCORES MEASURE:
       A. Daily fluctuations in depressed mood
       B. Relatively constant personality traits
       C. Moods which change within short time spans of a few minutes duration
       D. Vocational interests as opposed to vocational skills
       E. Motivation to perform in psychological experimentation
                                              Ref. 294 - p. 56

638.   MORUZZI HAS PROPOSED A CLASSIFICATION OF SLEEP:
       A. Based on the presence or absence of eye movements
       B. Based on a tonic-phasic dichotomy
       D. Which characterizes the sleep as good and poor sleep
       E. Which depends on the presence or absence of dream reports
                                              Ref. 294 - p. 56

639.   PONTINE-GENICULO-OCCIPITAL SPIKES (PGO SPIKES):
       A. Are monophasic discharges occurring during much of REM sleep
           and some parts of NREM sleep
       B. Relate to activity with the sustained inhibition of muscle tonus charac-
           teristic of REM
       C. Are associated with the sustained inhibition of muscle tonus charac-
           teristic of REM
       D. All of the above
       E. None of the above   Ref. 294 - p. 57

640.   SIGNIFICANT CORRELATION IS FOUND BETWEEN IMPROVEMENT OF
       DEPRESSION AND:
       A. Increase in REM sleep
       B. Decrease in stage 1
       C. Decrease in stage 4
       D. Decrease in phasic REM
       E. Decrease in sleep latency   Ref. 294 - p. 59

641. AFTER LONG-TERM TRENDS ARE PARTIALLED OUT, THE EEG
VARIABLE BEST CORRELATED WITH DAY-BY-DAY FLUCTUATIONS
IN DEPRESSIVE MOOD APPEARS TO BE:
A. REM percentage
B. Total time spent in REM sleep
C. Percentage of phasic REM
D. Sleep latency
E. Stage shifts   Ref. 294 - p. 59

642. PHENOMENA ASSOCIATED WITH PONTINE-GENICULO-OCCIPITAL
SPIKES INCLUDE THE FOLLOWING, EXCEPT:
A. Rapid eye movements
B. Bursts of automatic activity
C. General EEG activation of the REM stage
D. Muscle twitches
E. Saw-tooth waves in the EEG   Ref. 294 - p. 57

643. PRIMARY VISUAL EXPERIENCES:
A. Occur exclusively during REM sleep
B. Are tonic events
C. Are related to phasic events in REM and NREM sleep
D. Depend on mesencephalic reticular activity
E. Do not appear to be related to pontine reticular formation activity
Ref. 294 - p. 57

644. SECONDARY COGNITIVE ELABORATIONS:
A. Depend on PGO activity
B. Are characteristic of REM sleep
C. Are related to tonic phases of REM and NREM sleep
D. All of the above
E. None of the above   Ref. 294 - p. 57

645. THE LESS THE PERCENTAGE OF PHASIC REM DURING A NIGHT:
A. The less depression is complained of the next evening
B. The more patients complain the next evening of tiredness, loss of
appetite, and libido loss
C. The more the percentage of dream recall the next morning
D. The more vivid are the reported dreams
E. The more elated are the mood reports the next evening
Ref. 294 - p. 62

646. A SYNDROME FOUND IN INDIVIDUALS WITH A FAMILY HISTORY OF
ALLERGY AND CARBOHYDRATE-RELATED METABOLIC DISEASE,
WHICH APPEARS DUE IN PART TO UNKNOWN INTERMEDIATE METAB-
OLITES IN CERTAIN FOODS, HAS A MENTAL STATE CHARACTERIZED
BY:
A. Motor hyperactivity
B. Affective lability
C. Cognitive defects
D. All of the above
E. None of the above   Ref. 295 - p. 74

647. A DRUG WHICH HAS BEEN REPORTED TO HAVE REMEDIAL PROPER-
TIES IN CASES OF MULTIPLE TICS IS:
A. Thorazine
B. Valium
C. Lithium
D. Methysergide
E. Haloperidol   Ref. 296 - p. 79

648. COMPLEX TICS:
A. Carry psychological significance and appear to be expressions of
conflict over aggressive and sexual urges
B. Reflect a basis neurophysiological disorder with no psychological
meaning
C. Are unaffected by placebo
D. Have no resemblance to compulsive rituals
E. Are more prominent in the lower than upper limb
                                  Ref. 296 - p. 85

649. BRIEF PSYCHOTHERAPY WITH CHILDREN:
A. Should focus on the child without participation of the family because
of the limited amount of time available for treatment
B. Requires the development of rapport and positive transference
C. Works best when the issue of termination is dealt with one or two
sessions before treatment is ended
D. Cannot be effective if treatment is less than three months duration
E. Requires a passive approach on the therapist's part
                                  Ref. 297 - p. 143

650. BRIEF PSYCHOTHERAPY WITH CHILDREN IS HIGHLY EFFECTIVE:
A. When there is an ingredient of situational crisis
B. When there is a crisis involving object loss
C. For those therapists whose counteraggression problems make it
difficult for them to do long-term therapy
D. All of the above
E. None of the above   Ref. 297- p. 146

651. TO QUALIFY FOR REJECTION ON PSYCHIATRIC GROUNDS BY THE
SERVICE SYSTEM A DRAFT-ELIGIBLE MAN:
A. Must have a diagnosis of psychosis
B. Cannot have a diagnosis of psychoneurosis only
C. Cannot have a diagnosis of personality disorder only
D. All of the above
E. None of the above   Ref. 298 - p. 151

652. A PERSON WOULD BE REJECTED FROM MILITARY SERVICE IF HE
SUFFERED FROM:
A. A psychoneurotic reaction that caused prolonged care by a physician
(not psychoanalysis per se)
B. Overt homosexuality or other deviant sexual practices
C. Drug addiction
D. All of the above
E. None of the above   Ref. 298 - p. 151

102

653. THE EFFECT OF LITHIUM ON THYROID FUNCTION:
A. Is an antithyroid effect leading to frank hypothyroidism in some patients
B. Is to increase thyroid function and lead to hyperthyroidism in some patients
C. Is an increase in circulating thyroid hormone with an increase in uptake of iodine by the thyroid gland
D. Is the frequent development of thyroiditis
E. Is insignificant   Ref. 299 - p. 158

654. IT IS PROBABLE THAT AN ANTITHYROID EFFECT IS POSSESSED BY:
A. Imipramine
B. Chlorpromazine
C. Diazepam
D. Chlordiazepoxide
E. None of the above   Ref. 299 - p. 162

655. THERE IS A "SPOILING" NOTED OF THE ANTIMANIC EFFECT OF LITHIUM FOLLOWING THE ADDITION TO THE TREATMENT REGIMEN OF:
A. Sodium
B. Potassium
C. Haloperidol
D. Thyroid hormone
E. Insulin   Ref. 299 - p. 162

656. THE RUNAWAY REACTION:
A. Is a new diagnostic category in DSM-II
B. Is a result of compensatory overprotection by patients
C. Is best treated with brief psychotherapy and crisis intervention
D. Is rarely associated with stealing
E. Occurs in children who appear relatively mature for their age
Ref. 300 - p. 169

657. CHILDREN WHO ARE RESTLESS, INATTENTIVE, HAVE DIFFICULTY CONCENTRATING, SPEAK OUT OR JUMP OUT OF THEIR SEAT IN CLASS:
A. Are usually found to suffer from maternal deprivation
B. Generally come from minority groups
C. Probably suffer from the hyperkinetic syndrome
D. Should have Thorazine as the drug of choice
E. Show good adjustment in adult follow-up
Rèf. 301 - p. 177

658. CHILDREN WITH BEHAVIOR AND LEARNING DISORDERS SHOW GREATER IMPROVEMENT WITH DEXTROAMPHETAMINE TREATMENT:
A. When the drug is begun before age 5
B. If one or more neurological signs are present
C. With combined brief psychotherapy
D. When Thorazine is added to the treatment regimen
E. If the teacher can come to accept their behavior
Ref. 301 - p. 174

659. THE STANDARDIZED INTERVIEW DEVELOPED BY THE MEDICAL
RESEARCH COUNCIL AND THE UNITED STATES - UNITED KINGDOM
DIAGNOSTIC PROJECT IS THE:
A. Present State Examination
B. Mental Status Examination
C. Psychiatric Interview
D. Dynamic-Genetic Formulation
E. Free Association Interview   Ref. 302 - p. 180

660. ACUTE POSTOPERATIVE PSYCHOSES IN CHILDREN:
A. Are not expressed by hallucinatory activity
B. Are unaffected by the type of surgery
C. Have no relation to preoperative problems
D. All of the above
E. None of the above   Ref. 303 - p. 188

FOR QUESTIONS 661 - 672 SELECT THE LETTERED HEADING WHICH
BEST DESCRIBES THE MARIJUANA CHARACTERISTICS NOTED IN THE
1971 REPORT TO CONGRESS BY THE SECRETARY OF HEALTH,
EDUCATION AND WELFARE:

A. Impaired
B. Unchanged
C. Increased
D. Decreased
E. Inconsistent

661. ___ Sense of well-being
662. ___ Space perception
663. ___ Immediate memory
664. ___ Attention
665. ___ Sense of identity
666. ___ Suggestibility
667. ___ Hunger
668. ___ Predictability of drug effect when eating
669. ___ Pulse rate
670. ___ Pupil size
671. ___ Blood pressure
672. ___ Driving performance   Ref. 304 - p. 189-193

FOR EACH OF THE FOLLOWING MULTIPLE CHOICE QUESTIONS
SELECT THE MOST APPROPRIATE ANSWER:

673. MORTALITY STUDY OF PATIENTS SEEN IN A PSYCHIATRIC EMERGENC
ROOM REVEALS:
A. A death rate no higher than the general population
B. Alcoholism is a major cause of death
C. Suicide is the major cause of death
D. All of the above
E. None of the above   Ref. 305 - p. 223

104

674. GROUP ROUNDS IN A PSYCHIATRIC HOSPITAL ARE CHARACTERIZED BY THE FOLLOWING, EXCEPT:
A. Insure daily doctor-patient contact
B. Utilize observations of other patients
C. Poor acceptance by residents
D. Time-saving
E. Mutual patient support
Ref. 306 - p. 228

675. THE PRINCIPAL CHANGE IN THE EEG FOLLOWING SMOKING MARIJUANA IS:
A. Increase in percentage time alpha
B. Decrease in percentage time theta
C. Decrease in percentage time beta
D. All of the above
Ref. 307 - p. 196

676. A METHOD OF TIME ESTIMATION THAT DOES NOT APPEAR TO BE AFFECTED BY MARIJUANA IS:
A. True-false choice of interval
B. Multiple choice of interval
C. Reproduction of brief intervals
D. Free association estimation
E. None of the above
Ref. 307 - p. 195

677. IN CONTRAST TO HEAVY USERS, CASUAL USERS OF MARIJUANA:
A. Experience greater disruption of performance and perception
B. Do better on tests of performance
C. Describe a search for insight and a sense of harmony or union
D. Have a shorter duration of "high"
E. Have a greater sensitivity to the "high"
Ref. 308 - p. 202

678. DISTORTIONS IN TIME PERCEPTION WHILE UNDER THE INFLUENCE OF MARIJUANA:
A. Rarely occur in chronic users
B. Are more prominent when longer periods of time are being estimated
C. Occur under laboratory conditions but not in a social setting
D. Have not been demonstrated in the laboratory
E. Are self-correcting
Ref. 308 - p. 202

679. THE EFFECT OF MARIJUANA IN CHRONIC USERS MAY BE INFLUENCED BY:
A. Persisting levels of THC in the tissues over several days
B. Enzyme induction
C. The seeking of psychotomimetic effects by the user
D. All of the above
E. None of the above
Ref. 308 - p. 203

680. THE USE OF MARIJUANA BY U.S. SERVICEMEN IN VIET NAM:
A. Is complicated by admixture with opiates
B. Is associated with decreased incidence of disciplinary problems
C. Has diminished since 1965
D. Is condemned by the mental health personnel in the area
E. Is higher among officers
Ref. 309 - p. 204

681. A STUDY OF THE USE OF MARIJUANA IN FOUR WIDELY SEPARATED
      U.S. MEDICAL SCHOOLS REVEALED A:
      A. Lower incidence than found in high schools
      B. Lower incidence than found in colleges
      C. Lower incidence than found in soldiers in Viet Nam
      D. Higher incidence than found in soldiers in Viet Nam
      E. None of the above   Ref. 310 - p. 210

682. HALLUCINOGENIC EFFECTS OF MARIJUANA OCCUR ONLY:
      A. When other hallucinogens such as LSD or mescaline have been used
          previously
      B. When the drug has been used with great frequency
      C. In persons with pre-existent emotional disorder
      D. All of the above
      E. None of the above   Ref. 311 - p. 215

683. A FREQUENTLY REPORTED HALLUCINATION WHILE SMOKING
      MARIJUANA IS:
      A. Haptic
      B. Color
      C. Lilliputian
      D. Formication
      E. Blank   Ref. 311 - p. 215

684. MOBILIZATION OF HOSTILITY OUTWARD IN DEPRESSED PATIENTS:
      A. Is necessary for symptomatic improvement
      B. Has limited value and might be disastrous to tenuous relationships
      C. Is the goal of the psychotherapy of depression
      D. Is impaired since overt anger cannot be expressed
      E. Does not occur   Ref. 312 - p. 265

685. THE DEPRESSED PATIENT'S HOSTILITY:
      A. Is most manifest in initial rather than subsequent psychiatric interviews
      B. Is often not manifested during initial interviews
      C. Is directed more toward the physician rather than the nursing staff
          during hospital treatment
      D. Is directed toward the therapist only when the family is uninvolved
      E. Is rarely directed toward the therapist
                                               Ref. 312 - p. 265

686. THE OBJECT OF THE DEPRESSED PERSON'S GREATEST HOSTILITY
      IS THE:
      A. Spouse
      B. Parents
      C. Children
      D. Siblings
      E. Friend   Ref. 312 - p. 265

687. PERSONALITY TRAITS WHICH CARRY A POORER PROGNOSIS IN
      HOSPITAL-BASED DIALYSIS PATIENTS INCLUDE:
      A. Hyperindependence
      B. Recognition of illness
      C. Dependence
      D. Good pre-dialysis adaptation
      E. Compulsiveness   Ref. 313 - p. 272

688. A PREDICTOR OF SUCCESSFUL HOME DIALYSIS MAY BE:
    A. Denial of illness
    B. Impulsivity
    C. Hyperindependence
    D. All of the above
    E. None of the above   Ref. 313 - p. 272

689. IMPENDING DEATH MAY BE PREDICTED IN A PATIENT ON DIALYSIS WHEN:
    A. The wish to no longer live is expressed
    B. Suitable kidney for transplantation cannot be obtained
    C. More than two transplantations have ended in rejection
    D. Public funds become unavailable for maintenance of the dialysis program
    E. Family refuses donation of a suitably matching kidney
                                           Ref. 313 - p. 269

690. OBSERVATIONS OF ALCOHOLICS DURING PROLONGED DRINKING BOUTS REVEAL:
    A. Decreasing levels of tension and anxiety
    B. Improved mood and sociability
    C. Greater self-awareness
    D. Clinical evidence of profound depression
    E. Oceanic feelings   Ref. 314 - p. 275

691. THE CHRONIC ALCOHOLIC'S "DRINKING SYSTEM" IS:
    A. An open behavioral system
    B. A closed behavioral system
    C. A non-interactional system
    D. Unable to be categorized in systems theory
    E. None of the above   Ref. 314 - p. 279

692. THE ADVANTAGE OF DECISION ANALYSIS AS A BASIS FOR THE DECISION TO DISCHARGE A PATIENT FROM A MENTAL HOSPITAL IS:
    A. One aspect of the decision is emphasized to the exclusion of others
    B. All features are weighed equally
    C. Concern to avoid criticism for the decision is minimized
    D. All of the above
    E. None of the above   Ref. 315 - p. 285

693. IN THE DECISION ANALYSIS OF HOSPITAL DISCHARGE THE MOST UNDESIRABLE OUTCOME IS:
    A. Family complaints about release
    B. Patient dissatisfaction with decision
    C. Loneliness
    D. Dangerousness
    E. Indigency   Ref. 315 - p. 283

694. A FORM OF TREATMENT WHICH IS CONTRAINDICATED IN ANOREXIA NERVOSA IS:
    A. Intensive psychotherapy
    B. Behavior therapy
    C. Crisis-induced family therapy
    D. Hospitalization
    E. None of the above   Ref. 316 - p. 286

695. MORTALITY IN ANOREXIA NERVOSA IS AS HIGH AS:
  A. 100%
  B. 50%
  C. 15%
  D. 2%
  E. There is no mortality in this illness
  Ref. 316 - p. 286

696. THE PATUXENT INSTITUTE:
  A. Treats adolescent schizophrenics with long-term intensive psychotherapy
  B. Confines defective delinquents for an indeterminate sentence
  C. Was established for the treatment of heroin addiction by former addicts
  D. Has demonstrated success in the treatment of alcoholism
  E. Is a private institution in the treatment of adolescent heroin addicts
  Ref. 317 - p. 291

697. THE NATIONAL RATE OF RECIDIVISM OF PERSONS RELEASED FROM PRISON IS:
  A. 90%
  B. 70%
  C. 50%
  D. 30%
  E. 10%
  Ref. 317 - p. 293

698. HIGH MORNING RECALL OF DREAMS HAS BEEN RELATED TO THE PERSONALITY VARIABLE OF:
  A. Field independence
  B. High anxiety level
  C. Low ego strength
  D. Low repression
  E. All of the above
  Ref. 318 - p. 296

699. THE PARAMETER OF SLEEP PHYSIOLOGY THAT IS RELATED TO MORNING RECALL OF DREAMS IS:
  A. REM density
  B. Percentage of phasic REM
  C. REM latency
  D. Sleep latency
  E. Frequency of stage shifts
  Ref. 318 - p. 296

700. MORNING RECALL OF DREAMS IS FAVORED BY:
  A. Long consolidation time (time from night report to sleep onset)
  B. Position late in the night
  C. Short awakening reaction time
  D. All of the above
  E. None of the above
  Ref. 318 - p. 296

701. AN INDIVIDUAL DREAM IS LEAST LIKELY TO BE RECALLED WHEN IT IS THE:
  A. First dream in the night
  B. Second dream in the night
  C. Third dream in the night
  D. Fourth dream in the night
  E. Last dream in the night
  Ref. 318 - p. 298

702. A DREAM IS MORE LIKELY TO BE RECALLED WHEN IT IS:
   A. Short rather than long
   B. One of several reported during the night session
   C. Dramatically intense
   D. All of the above
   E. None of the above   Ref. 318 - p. 298

703. IT HAS BEEN DEMONSTRATED THAT THE DREAM CONTENT FAVORING
   MORNING RECALL IS PREDOMINANTLY:
   A. Sexual
   B. Aggressive
   C. Friendly
   D. Ambiguous
   E. No content variable favors dream recall
                                            Ref. 318 - p. 299

704. COMPARED TO THE ADOPTIVE FAMILIES, THE BIOLOGICAL
   FAMILIES OF ADOPTED SCHIZOPHRENICS SHOW:
   A. A higher prevalence of schizophrenia
   B. A lower prevalence of schizophrenia
   C. Similar prevalence of schizophrenia
   D. The comparison is meaningless because of the selective procedures
      of adoption agencies
   E. The comparison is meaningless because of the emotional instability
      of the mostly unmarried biological parents
                                            Ref. 319 - 1. 304

705. A STUDY OF THE TRANSMISSION OF SCHIZOPHRENIA USING ADOPTION
   AS A MEANS OF SEPARATION OF THE GENETIC AND ENVIRONMENTAL
   FACTORS:
   A. Does not separate these factors as well as twin studies do
   B. Avoids selective bias by the method of beginning with a total sample
      of adopted individuals
   C. Is unsatisfactory because of the higher incidence of schizophrenia
      in adopted individuals
   D. All of the above
   E. None of the above   Ref. 319 - p. 302

706. IN A GENETICALLY VULNERABLE INDIVIDUAL, A FACTOR WHICH
   MAY SERVE TO EVOKE A DISORDER IN THE SCHIZOPHRENIC SPECTRUM
   IS:
   A. Presence in the household of an individual who exhibits features of
      schizophrenia
   B. Child rearing practices
   C. Exposure to toxic or infectious agents
   D. Subtle personality characteristics
   E. All of the above   Ref. 319 - p. 304

707. NO DISORDERS IN THE SCHIZOPHRENIC SPECTRUM WERE FOUND IN
   THE BIOLOGICAL RELATIVES OF ADOPTED INDEX CASES DIAGNOSED
   AS:
   A. Acute schizophrenia
   B. Chronic schizophrenia
   C. Borderline schizophrenia
   D. All of the above
   E. None of the above   Ref. 319 - p. 305

708. THE ABOVE FINDING CALLS INTO QUESTION:
  A. The appropriateness if classifying acute psychotic reactions as schizophrenic disorders without further evidence from premorbid personality characteristics or the later course of the illness
  B. The entire concept of schizophrenia
  C. The usefulness of the borderline category
  D. The genetic basis of schizophrenia
  E. None of the above   Ref. 319 - p. 305

709. COMPARED TO SCHIZOPHRENIC WOMEN, SCHIZOPHRENIC MEN:
  A. Have more children
  B. Have fewer children
  C. Have the same number of children
  D. Can be more readily identified as the biological parents of adopted-away children
  E. None of the above   Ref. 320 - p. 308

710. THE ADOPTED-AWAY CHILDREN OF SCHIZOPHRENICS HAVE A RATE OF DIAGNOSIS OF SCHIZOPHRENIA WHICH IS:
  A. Lower than controls
  B. Equal to controls
  C. Higher than controls
  D. Higher than the children reared with their schizophrenic parents
  E. None of the above   Ref. 320 - p. 307

711. THE FOLLOWING ARE CATECHOLAMINES, EXCEPT:
  A. Dopamine
  B. Norepinephrine
  C. 3-methoxy, 4-hydroxy-mandelic acid (VMA)
  D. Tryptamine
  E. Metanephrine   Ref. 321 - p. 312

712. THE METABOLITE THAT IS CURRENTLY VIEWED AS PROVIDING THE MOST ACCURATE REFLECTION OF CNS CATECHOLAMINE METABOLISM IS:
  A. Normetanephrine
  B. VMA
  C. Dopamine
  D. 3-mehoxy, 4-hydroxy-phenylglycol (MHPG)
  E. Metanephrine   Ref. 321 - p. 315

713. A FINDING SUGGESTIVE OF AN ASSOCIATION WITH WHAT MAY LOOSELY BE TERMED THE "SCHIZOPHRENIC GENOTYPE" IS THAT MONOZYGOTIC TWINS DISCORDANT FOR SCHIZOPHRENIA BOTH HAVE ELEVATED URINARY LEVELS OF:
  A. Dopamine
  B. Norepinephrine
  C. Epinephrine
  D. Normetanephrine
  E. All of the above   Ref. 321 - p. 316

714. IT HAS BEEN SUGGESTED THAT A FINDING RELATED TO THE
SCHIZOPHRENIC PHENOTYPE IS AN ELEVATED LEVEL OF:
   A. 17-OH steroids
   B. MHPG
   C. Dopamine
   D. Norepinephrine
   E. All of the above   Ref. 321 - p. 316

715. THE POSSIBLE EXISTENCE OF A COMMON SUBSTRATE IN SCHIZO-
PHRENIA, PSYCHOTIC DEPRESSION, AND MANIA IS SUGGESTED BY
EACH DISORDER HAVING:
   A. Low levels of 17 OH steroids
   B. Low levels of catecholamines
   C. High levels of catecholamines
   D. High levels of indole amines
   E. Low levels of indole amines   Ref. 321 - p. 314

716. A NEW ANTIPSYCHOTIC AGENT, REPORTED TO BE AS EFFECTIVE
AS THE PHENOTHIAZINES, WHICH BLOCKS CNS DOPAMINE NEURONS
IS:
   A. Pimozide
   B. Methysergide
   C. Thiazide
   D. Aldomet
   E. Aldactone   Ref. 321 - p. 315

717. OF VALUE IN PREDICTING A POOR OUTCOME IN SCHIZOPHRENIA IS:
   A. Dyskinetic abnormal movements
   B. Hysterical features
   C. Depression
   D. All of the above
   E. None of the above   Ref. 322 - p. 318

718. TARDIVE DYSKINESIA IS ASSOCIATED WITH:
   A. Prolonged administration of neuroleptic drugs
   B. Organic brain lesions
   C. Old age
   D. All of the above
   E. None of the above   Ref. 322 - p. 317

719. PSYCHOSES WITH DYSKINETIC MOVEMENTS HAVE BEEN REPORTED
FOLLOWING TREATMENT WITH:
   A. Lithium
   B. L-dopa
   C. Pimozide
   D. Thiazide
   E. Magnesium   Ref. 322 - p. 321

720. THE GAP DESCRIPTION OF SCHIZOPHRENIFORM PSYCHOTIC DISORDER
IN CHILDREN IS CHARACTERIZED BY THE FOLLOWING, EXCEPT:
   A. Intensely independent of adults, especially the mother
   B. No evidence of psychosis during first six years of life
   C. Psychotic decompensation in early latency
   D. No crystallization into definite subtypes
   E. Relatively good prognosis   Ref. 323 - p. 324

721. HALLUCINATIONS IN CHILDREN WITH CHIZOPHRENIFORM PSYCHOSIS:
   A. Are not encountered
   B. Are rare before the age of nine
   C. Are auditory rather than visual
   D. Are not related to stress
   E. None of the above   Ref. 323 - p. 325

722. PSYCHOTHERAPY WITH CHILDREN WITH SCHIZOPHRENIFORM PSYCHOSIS:
   A. Is contraindicated
   B. Leads to intense positive attachments developing to the therapist
   C. Should always be combined with phenothiazine treatment
   D. Is more effective when not combined with tandem therapy for the mother
   E. Does not affect prognosis   Ref. 323 - p. 327

723. THE CORE SYMPTOMS IN SCHIZOPHRENIFORM PSYCHOSIS INCLUDE THE FOLLOWING, EXCEPT:
   A. Paranoid fantasies
   B. Paranoid peer relationships
   C. Difficulty distinguishing fantasies from reality
   D. Hallucinations
   E. Dyskinesias   Ref. 323 - p. 328

724. ACUTE CONFUSIONAL STATE IS FOUND IN:
   A. Psychoses of infancy
   B. Psychoses of early childhood
   C. Psychoses of later childhood
   D. Psychoses of adolescence
   E. None of the above   Ref. 323 - p. 330

725. IN SCHIZOAFFECTIVE DISORDER, THE AFFECT:
   A. Is flat
   B. Is inappropriate
   C. Is clearly one of depression or elation
   D. Of depression is capable of arousing an empathic reaction in those to whom the patient is close
   E. Is contagious   Ref. 324 - p. 334

FOR QUESTIONS 726 - 735, PAIR EACH CONCEPT WITH THE AUTHOR WITH WHOM IT IS IDENTIFIED:

    A. Kleist
    B. Gjessing
    C. Leonhard
    D. Langfeldt
    E. Winokur

726. ___ Thyrogenic catatonia
727. ___ Two types of schizoaffective psychoses
728. ___ Motility and confusion psychoses
729. ___ True schizophrenia and schizophreniform psychosis
730. ___ Cycloid or atypical psychosis

    A. Kraepelin
    B. Falret
    C. Morel
    D. Hecker
    E. Kahlbaum

731. ___ Demence precoce
732. ___ Hebephrenia
733. ___ Catatonia
734. ___ Manic-depressive psychosis
735. ___ Circular insanity   Ref. 324 - p. 333

SELECT THE MOST APPROPRIATE COMPLETION:

736. IN SCHIZOPHRENIA. THE AFFECT IS:
    A. Pure
    B. Congruent
    C. Contagious
    D. All of the above
    E. None of the above   Ref. 324 - p. 334

737. IN A PSYCHOSIS BROUGHT UNDER CONTROL, THE MOST IMPORTANT PREVENTIVE ELEMENT IS:
    A. ECT
    B. Maintenance drug therapy
    C. Insulin
    D. Age
    E. Milieu   Ref. 324 - p. 335

738. IN PATIENTS WITH INITIAL SCHIZOPHRENIC THOUGHT DISORDERS:
    A. The illness may shift to a predominantly affective one
    B. The prognosis is not affected by drug therapy
    C. ECT is contraindicated
    D. The course is constant rather than periodic
    E. Lithium is contraindicated   Ref. 324 - p. 335

739. IN CONTRAST TO SCHIZOPHRENICS WITHOUT THOUGHT PROCESS
DISORDER (TPD), SCHIZOPHRENICS WITH TPD REVEAL MORE OF THE
FOLLOWING, EXCEPT:
A. Sudden blocking
B. "Skidding" of one thought into another
C. Systematized delusions
D. Unsystematized delusions
E. Unintentional intrusions of primary process phenomena
Ref. 325 - p. 338

740. SCHIZOPHRENICS WITHOUT TPD MAY HAVE:
A. Histories of transient psychotic episodes
B. Coherent and focused thought pattern
C. Impoverishment of thinking
D. Thinking which is disorganized and bizarre
E. Systematized delusions   Ref. 325 - p. 338

741. SCHIZOPHRENICS WITH THOUGHT PROCESS DISORDERS REVEAL AN
AUDITORY EVOKED RESPONSE (AER) PATTERN WITH:
A. Similarity to the AER pattern of schizophrenics without TPD
B. Similarity in K complex amplitude
C. Similarity in K complex latency
D. High variability
E. Low variability   Ref. 325 - p. 338

742. EEG PERIOD ANALYSIS REVEALS THAT SCHIZOPHRENICS:
A. Have a greater amount of low voltage fast activity than normal
volunteers
B. Have a lesser amount of low voltage fast activity than normal
volunteers
C. With thought process disorder have a similar EEG pattern to those
without TPD
D. Without TPD have a greater amount of low voltage fast activity than
those with TPD
E. None of the above   Ref. 325 - p. 341

743. THE EEG OF SCHIZOPHRENICS SHOWS A:
A. High variability of amplitude
B. Low variability of amplitude
C. Contradictory finding in that variability of the electrical potential
as an auditory evoked response is high and variability of amplitude
is low
D. High amplitude
E. None of the above   Ref. 325 - p. 344

744. THE REACTION TO OUTSIDE STIMULI IS MODIFIED BY VARIATIONS
IN PERCEPTION AND INTERPRETATION:
A. In schizophrenia
B. Because of severe thought disorder
C. Which is a phenomenon associated with considerable variability in
the electrical potential of the auditory evoked response
D. All of the above
E. None of the above   Ref. 325 - p. 344

745. A HIGH MOLECULAR WEIGHT ALPHA GLOBULIN IS FOUND IN THE BLOOD PLASMA OF AT LEAST HALF THE PATIENTS WITH:
   A. Acute schizophrenia
   B. Chronic schizophrenia
   C. Depression
   D. Mania
   E. Hysteria   Ref. 326 - p. 348

746. AN EXAMPLE OF A PRIMARY PROCESS PHENOMENON IS:
   A. Translation of thought into visual imagery
   B. Bizarre way of thinking with condensation and displacement
   C. Loss of rules of time and space
   D. Mechanism of the dream work
   E. All of the above   Ref. 326 - p. 349

747. AN EFFECTIVE TREATMENT FOR THE TOXIC PSYCHOSIS OF LSD IS:
   A. VMA
   B. THC
   C. ECT
   D. MHPG
   E. None of the above   Ref. 327 - p. 352

748. THE EFFECT OF OBSERVATION ON THE THERAPEUTIC PROCESS IS:
   A. Minimal with the use of a one-way mirror
   B. To cause more obstacles and complications when the observer is in the treatment room compared to his beingbehind a one-way mirror
   C. Usually on the patient, but not on the therapist
   D. Usually on the therapist, but not on the patient
   E. None of the above   Ref. 328 - p. 355

749. COMPARABLE TO THE BEHAVIORIST CONCEPT OF DECREASE OR LACK IN POSITIVE REINFORCEMENT IS THE CONCEPT OF:
   A. The primary process
   B. Denial
   C. Identification with the aggressor
   D. Loss of object gratification
   E. Epigenesis   Ref. 329 - p. 358

750. THE ABOVE CONCEPTS HAVE RELEVANCE FOR:
   A. Schizophrenia
   B. Psychosis
   C. Prejudice
   D. Depression
   E. Maturation   Ref. 329 - p. 358

FOR QUESTIONS 751 - 758, MATCH THE CONCEPT WITH THE
AUTHOR WITH WHOM IT IS ASSOCIATED:

A. Loss or feared loss of an object of gratification resulting in depression
B. Loss of object leading to loss of self-esteem and ensuing depression
C. Frustration of needs and inability to achieve one's aspirations resulting in loss of self-esteem and feelings of depression
D. Depression, helplessness, and lack of self-esteem as reactions to frustrations and lack of gratification
E. Depression resulting from relative inability to acquire positive reinforcers

751. ___ Ferster
752. ___ Klein
753. ___ Rado
754. ___ Lazarus
755. ___ Jacobson
756. ___ Bibring
757. ___ Abraham
758. ___ Freud   Ref. 329 - pp. 358-359

SELECT THE MOST APPROPRIATE COMPLETION:

759. THE BASIC PRINCIPLE IN THE TREATMENT OF PSYCHIATRIC COMBAT CASUALITIES IS:
A. Immediacy
B. Proximity
C. Expectancy
D. Derived from the observations of Salmon on the English and French methods used in World War I
E. All of the above   Ref. 330 - p. 401

760. THE MOST IMPORTANT FUNCTIONS OF MILITARY PSYCHIATRY ARE:
A. Preventive
B. Draft counseling
C. Planning effective programs of psychological warfare
D. Improving morale in combat troops
E. All of the above   Ref. 330 - p. 401

761. THE CURRENT TREND IN MILITARY PSYCHIATRY IS:
A. Unit consultation
B. Development of peace movement programs
C. One-to-one treatment
D. Placement of the psychiatrist from the front lines to the rear
E. All of the above   Ref. 330 - p. 402

762. INDICATORS OF ORGANIZATIONAL STRESS IN THE MILITARY UNIT INCLUDE THE FOLLOWING, EXCEPT:
A. Requests for active duty
B. Venereal disease rates
C. Courts martial
D. Referrals for sick call
E. Article 15's   Ref. 330 - p. 402

116

763. THE CONCEPTUAL FRAMEWORK USED BY THE DEPARTMENT OF
INDUSTRIAL PSYCHIATRY AT THE MENNINGER FOUNDATION FOR THE
EVALUATION OF AN ORGANIZATION UTILIZES A POINT OF VIEW
WHICH IS:
A. Genetic
B. Economic
C. Topographic
D. Dynamic
E. All of the above   Ref. 330 - p. 402

764. A CENTRAL PHASE OF ORGANIZATIONAL CONSULTATION IN A MILITARY
COMBAT UNIT IS:
A. Use of a technician as a participant observer
B. Informal group meetings regarding use and dangers of hard drugs
C. Involvement of the unit commander in T group sessions
D. Venereal disease prevention program
E. All of the above   Ref. 330 - p. 403

765. A GROUP THAT WOULD BE CONSIDERED AT HIGH RISK FOR THE
DEVELOPMENT OF MENTAL ILLNESS IN A COMMUNITY HEALTH
CATCHMENT AREA IS:
A. Teen-aged mothers
B. Biracial marriages
C. Children of interracial couples
D. Widows
E. All of the above   Ref. 331 - p. 415

766. THE REPORT OF THE TASK FORCE ON JUVENILE DELINQUENCY OF
THE PRESIDENT'S COMMISSION ON LAW ENFORCEMENT AND THE
ADMINISTRATION OF JUSTICE:
A. Stresses internal psychological factors in the development of
delinquency
B. Recommends that counseling and therapy be made easily obtainable
C. Minimizes the role of the family structure in the etiology of delinquency
D. Points up the importance of military training in the reduction of
delinquency
E. All of the above   Ref. 332 - p. 421

767. THE FINAL REPORT OF THE PRESIDENT'S COMMISSION ON LAW
ENFORCEMENT AND THE ADMINISTRATION OF JUSTICE:
A. Recommends various kinds of psychological approaches for the
treatment of juvenile delinquency
B. Does not find that juvenile delinquency is related to poverty and
discrimination
C. Expresses disagreement with the Task Force Report on Juvenile
Delinquency
D. Recommends strengthening the system of juvenile justice
E. Stresses internal psychological problems as the basis of juvenile
delinquency   Ref. 332 - p. 421

768. ACCORDING TO SLAVSON, THE "DOOM MOTIF" IS:
A. Often a self-fulfilling prophecy
B. An extension of the delinquent's parents' punitive and denigrating
attitudes toward him
C. An unspoken appeal to be rescued
D. All of the above
E. None of the above   Ref. 332 - p. 421

769. THE AWARENESS BY DELINQUENTS OF THEIR OWN IMPULSIVITY IS
     RELATED TO:
     A. Age
     B. Race
     C. Objective measures of impulsivity
     D. Race
     E. Police contact   Ref. 332 - p. 421

770. THE NATIONAL COMMISSION ON THE CAUSES AND PREVENTION OF
     VIOLENCE:
     A. Was impanelled following the assassination of John Kennedy
     B. Was the first presidential commission, established in response to a
        political crisis, that included a psychiatrist
     C. Contained a majority of behavioral scientists
     D. All of the above
     E. None of the above   Ref. 333 - p. 431

771. THE FOCUS OF THE VIOLENCE COMMISSION WAS ON:
     A. Evironmental problems that were causative factors in violence
     B. Individual personality characteristics that contribute to the problem
        of violence
     C. Recommendations for action by individual citizens
     D. Strengthening law and order
     E. Changing existing laws   Ref. 333 - p. 434

772. ACCORDING TO LORENZ, THE GREATEST AMOUNT OF FIGHTING IS
     FOUND IN SPECIES WHOSE SOCIAL ORGANIZATION:
     A. Includes a definite bond between individuals
     B. Is characterized by the formation of groups
     C. Is that of an anonymous crowd
     D. Is fluid rather than stable
     E. Undergoes rapid change   Ref. 334 - p. 436

773. THE SHORTEST PERCENTAGE OF LIFESPAN SPENT IN A PERIOD OF
     INFANT DEPENDENCY ON THE MOTHER IS FOUND IN:
     A. Man
     B. Chimpanzee
     C. Gorilla
     D. Baboon
     E. Rhesus monkey   Ref. 334 - p. 437

774. THE PERCENTAGE OF THE LIFESPAN SPENT IN THE STATE MARKED
     BY CLOSENESS CHARACTERISTIC TO THE PERIOD OF INFANT
     DEPENDENCY ON THE MOTHER CORRELATES WELL WITH:
     A. Resistance to disease
     B. Affectional bonding in primates
     C. Rapidity of neuromuscular maturation
     D. Emotional disorder
     E. Depressive diathesis   Ref. 334 - p. 437

775. THE SOCIAL AND CULTURAL PATTERN IN TAHITI IS CHARACTERIZED
BY THE FOLLOWING, EXCEPT:
A. High rate of adoption
B. Fragile and conditional relationships between parent and children
C. Elaborately organized religion
D. Limitations in the related characteristics of spontaneity and creativity
E. No written language   Ref. 334 - p. 440

FOR QUESTIONS 776 - 805, ONE OR MORE OF THE COMPLETIONS
IS CORRECT. SELECT:

A. If only 1, 2, and 3 are correct
B. If only 1 and 3 are correct
C. If only 2 and 4 are correct
D. If only 4 is correct
E. If all are correct

776. CULTURES WITH HIGH SYNERGY (BENEDICT):
1. Provide for acts that are mutually reinforcing
2. Have conspicuous nonaggression
3. Have social orders in which the individual by the same act serves
his own advantage and that of the group
4. Have social situations which provide for acts that are mutually opposed
and counteractive   Ref. 334 - p. 443

777. CULTURES WHICH ARE CHARACTERIZED BY MUCH AGGRESSION,
ANXIETY, AND LOW MORALE INCLUDE THE:
1. Chuckchee
2. Ojibwa
3. Dobu
4. Kwakiutl   Ref. 334 - p. 443

778. CULTURES WHICH ARE CHARACTERIZED BY AFFECTION, SECURITY,
AND NONAGGRESSION INCLUDE THE:
1. Dakota
2. Arapesh
3. Zuni
4. Kwakiutl   Ref. 334 - p. 443

779. HIGH INTENSITY INTERPERSONAL BONDING APPEARS TO BE A
PREREQUISITE FOR:
1. Cultural achievement
2. Aggressive behavior
3. Mental illness
4. Security   Ref. 334 - p. 436

780. REDUCTION OF AGGRESSION AND MENTAL ILLNESS, WHILE MAIN-
TAINING A HIGH LEVEL OF CULTURAL ACHIEVEMENT MAY BE
BROUGHT ABOUT BY:
1. Increasing areas of productive competition
2. Increasing interpersonal intensity within the family
3. Increasing social mobility
4. Increasing synergy   Ref. 334 - p. 436

781. MOST OF THE CHILDREN IN THE EXPERIENTIALLY DETERMINED
SCHOOL LEARNING DISABILITY POPULATION COME FROM GROUPS
IN SOCIETY THAT ARE:
1. Deprived economically
2. The objects of prejudice
3. The victims of aggression
4. Socially mobile   Ref. 335 - p. 446

782. ACCORDING TO GEORGE GARDNER, THE GREATEST STRUGGLE OF
MAN IS THE STRUGGLE TO CONTROL:
1. Sexual impulses
2. Prejudice
3. Pollution of the environment
4. Violence   Ref. 335 - p. 445

783. OBSERVATIONS OF PRECISION LEARNING DISABILITY CHILDREN
INDICATE THAT AN APPRECIABLE NUMBER OF SUCH CASES CARRY
AN EXTREME OVERLOAD OF ANXIETY ARISING FROM:
1. An excess of traumatic incidents during the first six years of life
2. Frequent moves by the family
3. Violent events in their first six years
4. Family pressure to compete and succeed
                                      Ref. 335 - p. 448

784. THE DEFENSE UTILIZED BY THE CHILD WITH PRECISION LEARNING
DISABILITY TO CONTROL FEAR ELICITED BY THE PRESENTATION
OF PROBLEM-SOLVING SITUATIONS IS:
1. Withdrawal into fantasy
2. Overactivity
3. Attention to distracting items in the environment
4. Stimulation and utilization of peers to effect distracting events
                                      Ref. 335 - p. 450

785. THE OCCURRENCE OF SLAUGHTER OF DEFENSELESS VICTIMS IN
WAR IS RELATED TO:
1. Dilution of responsibility
2. Dehumanization of the enemy
3. Universalization of the enemy
4. Natural dominance of the psychopath in war
                                      Ref. 336 - p. 451

786. THOSE INVOLVED IN THE SLAUGHTER OF DEFENSELESS VICTIMS
IN WAR:
1. Often do not experience guilt
2. Are generally psychopathic
3. Often feel profound guilt
4. Rarely use drugs   Ref. 336 - p. 451

787. A PHENOMENON WHICH NECESSARILY INVOLVES DESTRUCTIVENES
IS:
1. Hate
2. Violence
3. Hostility
4. Anger   Ref. 337 - p. 456

788. FOR HUMANS, AN ALERTING PHENOMENON FOR THE INDIVIDUAL AND FOR OTHERS THAT PROVIDES A BASIS FOR COMMUNICATION IS:
1. Hate
2. Violence
3. Hostility
4. Anger
Ref. 337 - p. 457

789. HOSTILITY:
1. Allows the object to remove particular threats or obstructions
2. Tends to destroy the object itself
3. May be related to basic respect for a loved person
4. May be manifested by sarcasm, teasing, gossip, and passive obstructiveness
Ref. 337 - p. 457

790. VIOLENCE OCCURS WHEN:
1. Motoric arousal is undirected or directed toward avoidance or escape
2. Anger cannot serve as a sufficient alerting process
3. Motoric arousal begins to be directed at the source of threat or obstruction
4. Anger is unexpressed and threats cannot be removed
Ref. 337 - p. 459

791. THE MOST TRULY VIOLENT PEOPLE ARE THOSE WHO:
1. Express anger freely
2. Have no guilt about angry feelings
3. Defend against anxiety with anger
4. Have difficulty dealing with angry feelings
Ref. 337 - p. 460

792. ADOLESCENTS WHO COMMIT HOMICIDE FREQUENTLY HAVE PRO-DROMAL SIGNS WHICH INCLUDE:
1. Mood shifts, especially toward pessimism
2. A "call for help" that is not perceived by those in daily contact with the adolescent
3. Use of drugs
4. Somatization
Ref. 338 - p. 461

793. HOMICIDES IN ADOLESCENTS ARE OFTEN PRECIPITATED BY:
1. Psychotherapeutic intervention
2. Threats to manhood
3. Lack of scholastic achievement
4. Homosexual threats
Ref. 338 - p. 464

794. ON A FREQUENT FIXED-INTERVAL-DRINKING-DECISIONS (FIDD) RESEARCH MODEL, ALCOHOLICS:
1. Usually take all the drinks available
2. May take no drinks at all
3. Rarely cooperate to complete the experiment
4. Who are nondrinkers emerge as leaders of the group
Ref. 339 - p. 478

795. THE CONTRIBUTION OF MENDELSON AND HIS COWORKERS IN THE STUDY OF ALCOHOLISM IS:
    1. Experimentally induced inebriation
    2. Treatment of alcoholics by intensive psychotherapy
    3. Giving alcohol to the alcoholic under controlled conditions
    4. Treatment of alcoholism by LSD   Ref. 339 - p. 475

796. THE ADMINISTRATION OF IMIPRAMINE ON A ONCE A DAY BASIS IS:
    1. Less efficient therapeutically
    2. Associated with undesirable side effects, especially insomnia
    3. Associated with abnormal liver function tests
    4. More convenient for the nursing staff
                                            Ref. 340 - p. 484

797. GILLES DE LA TOURETTE'S SYNDROME CONSISTS OF:
    1. Facial tics and grimacing
    2. Explosive involuntary movement of neck, shoulders, trunk, and legs
    3. Loud expiratory grunts and barks
    4. Echolalia and coprolalia   Ref. 341 - p. 491

798. MAXWELL JONES' GOAL FOR A THERAPEUTIC COMMUNITY IS:
    1. Active treatment
    2. Democracy
    3. Permissiveness
    4. Less specialized staff roles   Ref. 342 - p. 492

799. AN ECT INSTRUMENT IN COMMON USE IS THE:
    1. Reuben Reiter MOL-AC II
    2. Tektronix RM564
    3. Medcraft Model B24
    4. Tektronix P6006   Ref. 343 - p. 97

800. THE GLISSANDO MODE OF ECT USE:
    1. Was ostensibly introduced to provide slower onset of seizure and thereby reduce bone fractures
    2. May unduly prolong the duration of ECT
    3. Is not conclusively effective
    4. Is especially useful when combined with succinylcholine
                                            Ref. 343 - p. 99

801. AN ECT INSTRUMENT SHOULD BE PROVIDED WITH:
    1. Automatic regulation of voltage
    2. Automatic regulation of impulse duration
    3. Accurate manufacturer's specifications
    4. Glissando mode   Ref. 343 - p. 99

802. THE LEGAL GROUNDS ON WHICH A PATIENT MAY RELY IN PRESSING A SUIT RELATING TO ECT USE ARE:
    1. No consent for the treatment
    2. Failure to use muscle relaxant
    3. Failure to have facilities available for management of cardiorespiratory emergencies occurring during ECT
    4. Failure to use ECT where indicated
                                            Ref. 344 - p. 101

803. THE USE OF MUSCLE RELAXANTS AND ANESTHESIA INCREASE THE RISK OF:
1. Cardiac arrhythmias
2. Hypotension
3. Aspiration pneumonia
4. Agranulocytosis   Ref. 344 - p. 101

804. RISK-MARKERS WHICH OCCUR MORE FREQUENTLY IN HOSPITALIZED PATIENTS THAN IN THE GENERAL POPULATION INCLUDE:
1. Divorce or separation
2. Family member beginning heavy drinking
3. Trouble with the police
4. Onset of heavy drinking   Ref. 345 - p. 106

805. RISK-MARKERS WHICH MIGHT BE USEFUL IN A PROGRAM OF PRIMARY PREVENTION INCLUDE:
1. Divorce/separation
2. Development of problem drinking
3. Onset of alcohol abuse in an immediate family member
4. Being in trouble with the police   Ref. 345 - p. 108

SELECT THE MOST APPROPRIATE ANSWER FOR THE FOLLOWING MULTIPLE CHOICE QUESTIONS:

806. THE OVERALL PATTERN OF DIAGNOSTIC DIFFERENCES BETWEEN AMERICAN AND BRITISH PSYCHIATRISTS INDICATES THAT:
A. The American concept of schizophrenia is much broader than the British concept
B. There is a greater influence of psychoanalytic thinking in the United Kingdom
C. Americans are more prone to use the term "hysteria" than their British counterparts
D. British thinking is more in line with the usage on the East Coast of the United States compared to the Mid-West and West
E. The British rarely use the manic-depressive category
                                            Ref. 346 - p. 129

807. THE 1968 TABLES OF FIRST ADMISSIONS TO THE PUBLIC MENTAL HOSPITALS COMPILED BY THE BIOMETRY BRANCH OF THE NIMH SHOW THAT:
A. The prevalence of schizophrenia is higher on the West Coast than the East Coast
B. The prevalence of schizophrenia is higher in the South compared to the rest of the country
C. Half of the admissions in New York State other than organic brain syndromes and addictive states are diagnosed as schizophrenics
D. Half of the admissions in California other than organic brain syndromes and addictive states are diagnosed as schizophrenics
E. All of the above   Ref. 346 - p. 130

808. THE DIAGNOSIS OF MANIA IS:
  A. No longer used in Britain
  B. Used with greater frequency since the introduction of lithium as a specific treatment
  C. In danger of disappearing now from usage in the United States
  D. Used with greater frequency since the introduction of chlorpromazine
  E. None of the above   Ref. 346 - p. 129

809. THE HYSTERICAL PERSONALITY IS CHARACTERIZED BY THE FOLLOWING, EXCEPT:
  A. Excitability
  B. Parsimoniousness
  C. Self-dramatization
  D. Immaturity
  E. Unusual dependence   Ref. 347 - p. 131

810. THE HEALTHY HYSTERIC IN CONTRAST TO THE SICK HYSTERIC IS MORE LIKELY TO:
  A. Be sexually promiscuous
  B. Experience little guilt
  C. Be the father's favorite
  D. Have no genuine period of latency
  E. Devalue her femininity   Ref. 347 - p. 135

811. THE SICK HYSTERIC, IN CONTRAST TO THE HEALTHY HYSTERIC:
  A. Shows a predominance of oedipal conflicts over oral ones
  B. Has presenting problems revolving in the main around sexual behavior and the real or fantasied sexual object
  C. Utilizes against passivity and orality
  E. Is ambitious and competitive   Ref. 347 - p. 135

812. IN THE HISTORICAL DEVELOPMENT OF GENERAL PSYCHIATRY OUTSIDE OF PSYCHOANALYTIC CIRCLES, AND IN DSM-II, HYSTERIA AND THE HYSTERICAL CHARACTER REFER TO PATIENTS WITH:
  A. Gross symptoms
  B. Gross character traits
  C. Major ego disturbances
  D. All of the above
  E. None of the above   Ref. 347 - p. 136

813. THE USEFULNESS OF AMPHETAMINES IN CHILDREN WITH BEHAVIOR DISORDERS APPEARS TO BE LIMITED BY:
  A. Presence or absence of overt anxiety
  B. Presence or absence of hyperactivity
  C. Presence or absence of minimal brain damage
  D. Intensity of psychomotor excitement
  E. All of the above   Ref. 348 - p. 197

814. CLINICAL GROUPS WHICH RESPOND POORLY TO AMPHETAMINES INCLUDE:
  A. Overtly psychotic schizophrenic children
  B. Children with grossly psychotic symptoms
  C. Children who manifest severely impulsive, forceful and disorganized hyperactivity with little external provocation
  D. Children with behavior disorders severe enough to necessitate hospitalization
  E. All of the above   Ref. 348 - p. 195

815. CHILDREN REPORTED AS RESPONDING TO AMPHETAMINES INCLUDE
THOSE WITH PREDOMINANCE OF:
A. Anxiety
B. Neurotic mechanisms
C. Negativism
D. Belligerence
E. All of the above   Ref. 348 - p. 197

816. CHILDREN WHO IN THE DSM-II WOULD BE DIAGNOSED AS "OVER-
ANXIOUS REACTION" AND "UNSOCIALIZED AGGRESSIVE REACTION"
RESPOND TO AMPHETAMINES ONLY WHEN THERE IS ASSOCIATED:
A. Hyperactive state
B. Mental retardation
C. Organic brain syndrome
D. All of the above
E. None of the above   Ref. 348 - p. 197

817. FOR THE DIAGNOSIS OF SCHIZOPHRENIA IN CHILDREN NECESSARY
SYMPTOMS ARE:
A. Autism and thought disorder
B. Affect severely underresponsive
C. Mutism and confusion regarding personal identity
D. Dyskinetic motility
E. All of the above   Ref. 348 - p. 201

818. AUTISM CONSISTS OF THE FOLLOWING, EXCEPT:
A. Little or bizarre human interaction
B. Defiance, hostility, and belligerence
C. Extreme preoccupation with internal stimuli
D. Response which appears dictated by inner impulses and experiences,
   and which appears inappropriate to external stimuli
E. Gross impairment of relationships with people and the environment
                                       Ref. 348 - p. 201

819. THE DIAGNOSTIC CATEGORY OF UNSOCIALIZED AGGRESSIVE
REACTION IN CHILDREN COMMONLY SHOWS:
A. Psychosis
B. Poorly integrated and generally inadequate behavior
C. Denial of anxiety
D. Sadness
E. Group delinquent reaction   Ref. 348 - p. 202

820. THE DIAGNOSIS OF OVERANXIOUS REACTION AND WITHDRAWING
REACTION IN CHILDREN IS DISQUALIFIED BY THE PRESENCE OF THE
FOLLOWING, EXCEPT:
A. Compliance
B. Psychosis
C. Hostility
D. Denial of sadness
E. Denial of anxiety   Ref. 348 - p. 202

821. A DRUG WHICH HAS BEEN REPORTED TO BE EFFECTIVE IN BLOCKING
PANIC ATTACKS IN AGORAPHOBIC ADULTS IS:
   A. Methylphenidate
   B. Diphenhydramine
   C. Imipramine
   D. Dextroamphetamine
   E. Diphenylhydantion   Ref. 349 - p. 204

822. THE ABOVE DRUG HAS BEEN REPORTED TO BE SIGNIFICANTLY
SUPERIOR TO PLACEBO IN THE TREATMENT IN CHILDREN OF:
   A. Hyperactive reaction
   B. Unsocialized aggressive reaction
   C. Overanxious reaction
   D. School phobia
   E. Withdrawal reaction   Ref. 349 - p. 205

823. NECESSARY INGREDIENTS FOR THE DOUBLE-BIND SITUATION INCLUDE
THE FOLLOWING, EXCEPT:
   A. Primary negative injunction
   B. Secondary injunction confliction with the first at a more abstract level
   C. Tertiary negative injunction prohibiting escape from the field
   D. Repeated experience
   E. Three or more persons   Ref. 350 - p. 233

824. WITH THE TACHISTOSCOPIC PRESENTATION OF RORSCHACH CARDS,
THE BRIEFEST EXPOSURES RESULT IN:
   A. Abstract responses
   B. Responses resembling those of a child
   C. Position responses
   D. Movement responses
   E. No responses   Ref. 350 - p. 235

825. A CHILD'S SECURITY BLANKET CORRESPONDS ROUGHLY TO THE
CONCEPT OF:
   A. Anaclitic love object
   B. Narcissistic love object
   C. Transitional object
   D. Imago
   E. Autism   Ref. 350 - p. 236

826. THERE IS A BETTER PROGNOSIS FOR A THERAPEUTIC RESPONSE
TO TRICYCLIC ANTIDEPRESSANTS IN PATIENTS WHO:
   A. Manifest an early autonomic response
   B. Do not experience sweating
   C. Have a rise in systolic blood pressure
   D. Have a reactive rather than endogenous depression
   E. Have a history of suicide attempts   Ref. 351 - p. 247

827. THERE IS SOME EVIDENCE THAT A THERAPEUTIC RESPONSE TO
TRICYCLIC ANTIDEPRESSANTS MAY BE PREDICTED BY A POSITIVE
RESPONSE TO:
   A. Cannabis
   B. Dextroamphetamine
   C. Diphenylhydantion
   D. Thyroid hormone
   E. LSD   Ref. 351 - p. 254

828. A FALL IN PLASMA HUMAN GROWTH HORMONE OCCURS:
A. Following a fall in blood glucose concentration
B. In states of emotional arousal
C. During deep slow-wave sleep
D. All of the above
E. None of the above   Ref. 352 - p. 263

829. HUMAN GROWTH HORMONE RESPONSES TO INSULIN TOLERANCE TESTS ARE OFTEN DEFICIENT:
A. In children with the maternal deprivation syndrome
B. During depression
C. Following recovery from depression
D. All of the above
E. None of the above   Ref. 352 - p. 263

830. THE MANIC PATIENT'S PLASMA CORTISOL LEVELS:
A. Are elevated during the evening
B. Show a loss of diurnal rhythm
C. Suggest that psychological defenses are less effective during the day
D. All of the above
E. None of the above   Ref. 353 - p. 272

831. THE SLEEP PATTERN IN A HYPOMANIC PATIENT AS MEASURED BY THE EEG SHOWS AN INCREASED:
A. Total sleep time
B. Actual sleep time
C. REM
D. All of the above
E. None of the above   Ref. 354 - p. 276

832. THE TENDENCY OF NARCOTIC ADDICTS TO FORM AN ANTITHERA-PEUTIC COMMUNITY CAN BE MINIMIZED BY:
A. Treatment of the addict in a general psychiatric ward
B. Separation of addicts in isolated psychiatric wards
C. Development of an ex-addict staff parallel to the nursing staff
D. Use of chlorpromazine in high doses
E. Use of methadone for detoxification
          Ref. 355 - p. 283

833. PENTYLENETETRAZOL, PAPAVERINE, AND NIACIN HAVE BEEN USED FOR THE TREATMENT OF:
A. Epilepsy
B. Heroin addiction
C. Hyperactivity in children
D. Senile brain disorders
E. Mania   Ref. 356 - p. 284

834. THE GEMEINSCHAFT COMMUNITY:
A. Is characteristic of urban industrial societies
B. Has formal and explicit bonds
C. Operates on the basis of mutual dependence of individual members
D. Has formal rules of relationship
E. Is exemplified by civic organizations
          Ref. 357 - p. 291

835.   THE GESELLSCHAFT COMMUNITY:
    A. Is like the extended family
    B. Becomes increasingly rare
    C. Is held together by common values and affection
    D. Utilizes formulated guidelines and rules for relationships
    E. Depends for its existence on rural social organization
                           Ref. 357 - p. 291

836.   AN EXAMPLE OF A GEMEINSCHAFT COMMUNITY IS THE:
    A. Democratic party
    B. Amish
    C. Teamsters Union
    D. American Medical Association
    E. Catholic Church   Ref. 357 - p. 292

837.   THE FAMILY IS A COMMUNITY WHICH IN TYPE IS:
    A. Gemeinschaft
    B. Gesellschaft
    C. Franchiser
    D. All of the above
    E. None of the above   Ref. 357 - p. 292

838.   WHITEHORN AND BETTS' TYPE A THERAPISTS ARE THREE TIMES AS
    SUCCESSFUL AS TYPE B THERAPISTS IN ELICITING IMPROVEMENT IN:
    A. Schizophrenic patients
    B. Depressive patients
    C. Neurotic patients
    D. All of the above
    E. None of the above   Ref. 358 - p. 303

839.   TYPE A THERAPISTS:
    A. Have treatment goals defined in terms of eliminating symptomatology
    B. Are located towards the directive end of the therapeutic spectrum
    C. Are more interested in the psychopathology of the patient rather than
        in his personality
    D. Are actively involved in their relationships with the patient
    E. Do poorly with neurotic patients   Ref. 358 - p. 303

840.   IN THE INTRODUCTORY LECTURES, FREUD DEFINES THE CATEGORY
    OF ANXIETY WHICH IS A REACTION TO EXTERNAL DANGER AS:
    A. Expectant anxiety
    B. Bound anxiety
    C. Free-floating anxiety
    D. Actual anxiety
    E. Stranger anxiety   Ref. 358 - p. 301

841.   IN THE PROBLEM OF ANXIETY, FREUD STATES THAT ANXIETY:
    A. Arises in the id
    B. Follows repression
    C. Precedes repression
    D. Is unrelated to repression
    E. Is unrelated to castration fantasies
                          Ref. 358 - p. 301

842.   THE USE OF THE COUCH IN THE PSYCHOTHERAPY OF BORDERLINE
        PATIENTS:
        A.   Should be limited to skilled and experienced therapists
        B.   May be attempted cautiously by beginning therapists
        C.   Satisfies affect hunger
        D.   Does not foster regression
        E.   Encourages autonomy in the patient   Ref. 359 - p. 313

843.   IN THE AVOIDANCE CONDITIONING TECHNIQUE FOR THE TREATMENT
        OF HOMOSEXUAL MEN THE FOLLOWING ARE EMPLOYED, EXCEPT:
        A.   Pictures of men
        B.   Pictures of women
        C.   Painful electric shocks
        D.   Sedation
        E.   Response keys   Ref. 360 - p. 314

844.   THE AVOIDANCE CONDITIONING TREATMENT OF HOMOSEXUALITY
        IN MEN:
        A.   Results in extinction of homosexual responses
        B.   Leads to suppression of homosexual responses through punishment
        C.   Works behaviorally even if punishment is not continued
        D.   Is not helped by concomitant psychotherapy
        E.   Has results no different from placebo
                                                     Ref. 360 - p. 323

845.   A PROGRAM FOR A COMPUTER-CONTROLLED PSYCHOTHERAPEUTIC
        INTERVIEW WHICH TAKES AFFECTIVE RESPONSES INTO ACCOUNT
        IS KNOWN AS:
        A.   Therapy
        B.   Insight
        C.   Affect
        D.   PL/ACME
        E.   360/50   Ref. 361 - p. 324

846.   OF THE FOLLOWING LIFE STRESS EVENTS, THE ONE WHICH CAUSES
        THE GREATEST UPSET APPEARS TO BE:
        A.   Death of child
        B.   Divorce
        C.   Miscarriage
        D.   Menopause
        E.   Business failure   Ref. 362 - p. 341

847.   ACTIVITY OF RED BLOOD CELL CATECHOL-O-METHYLTRANSFERASE
        (COMT) IS LOWER IN WOMEN WITH:
        A.   Primary affective disorder
        B.   Schizophrenia
        C.   Antisocial personality
        D.   All of the above
        E.   None of the above   Ref. 363 - p. 348

848.   FACTORS WHICH DIFFERENTIATE AFFECTIVELY ILL MEN AND WOMEN
        INCLUDE:
        A.   Red blood cell indices
        B.   Enhancement of antidepressant action of imipramine by thyroid hormone
        C.   Degree of depression
        D.   Lithium response
        E.   All of the above   Ref. 363 - p. 352

IN QUESTIONS 849 - 858, MATCH EACH LETTERED DEPRESSIVE CATEGORY WITH THE ASSOCIATED CLINICAL AND BIOLOGICAL PARAMETERS:

A. Unipolar
B. Bipolar
C. Both unipolar and bipolar
D. Neither unipolar nor bipolar

849. ___ More pacing behavior, overt anger, and physical complaints
850. ___ Production of hypomania and mania by Levodopa
851. ___ Mild to moderate antidepressant effect of lithium carbonate
852. ___ Elevation of plasma magnesium in response to lithium carbonate administration
853. ___ Lower threshold to flicker stimulation
854. ___ Augmenting pattern of evoked cortical response
855. ___ Reduced urinary excretion of 17-hydroxycorticosteroids
856. ___ Elevated COMT activity
857. ___ Lowest COMT activity
858. ___ Deficiency of catecholamines at functionally important neural receptors
Ref. 363 - pp. 348,350,352

FOR EACH OF THE FOLLOWING MULTIPLE CHOICE QUESTIONS SELECT THE MOST APPROPRIATE ANSWER:

859. NOREPINEPHRINE REUPTAKE AT NORADRENERGIC NEURONS IS INHIBITED BY:
A. Reserpine
B. Amitriptyline
C. Imipramine
D. All of the above
E. None of the above   Ref. 363 - p. 351

860. IN THE CSF OF PATIENTS WITH ENDOGENOUS DEPRESSIONS:
A. The metabolite of dopamine, homovanillic acid (HVA), is decreased
B. The metabolite of serotonin, 5-hydroxyindoleacetic acid (5-HIAA), is decreased
C. 5-HIAA is decreased following treatment with imipramine
D. 5-HIAA is decreased following treatment with amitriptyline
E. All of the above   Ref. 364 - p. 357

861. THE RESULT OF IMIPRAMINE TREATMENT ON THE CSF CONCENTRATION OF 5-HIAA COMES ABOUT BY:
A. Inhibition of serotonin (5-HT) reuptake mechanisms by imipramine
B. Decreased intracellular deamination caused by decreased reuptake
C. Decreased 5-HIAA formation intracellularly because of decreased deamination
D. All of the above
E. None of the above   Ref. 364 - p. 357

862. THE EFFECT OF IMIPRAMINE ON THE CSF CONCENTRATION OF HVA
IS:
A. Increased concentration because of increased dopamine reuptake in the caudate nucleus
B. Decreased concentration because of increased dopamine reuptake in the caudate nucleus
C. Unchanged because dopamine reuptake in the caudate nucleus does not appear to be sensitive to imipramine
D. Increased because of decreased dopamine reuptake in the caudate nucleus
E. Decreased because of decreased dopamine reuptake in the caudate nucleus
Ref. 364 - p. 357

863. ALTHOUGH THE 8 AM TYROSINE PLASMA CONCENTRATION IS ABOUT EQUAL, THERE IS A SIGNIFICANT DECREASE IN THE 11 AM CONCENTRATION IN:
A. Schizophrenics
B. Endogenous depressives
C. Neurotic depressives
D. Healthy controls
E. All of the above
Ref. 365 - p. 359

864. IN DREAMS, THERE IS A PRONOUNCED SHIFT TOWARD MORE NOVELTY:
A. Earlier than later in the night
B. In men rather than in women
C. In the overall dream than in the constituent elements of the dream
D. All of the above
E. None of the above
Ref. 366 - p. 368

865. THE MOST POTENT INHIBITORS OF REM SLEEP DISCOVERED THUS FAR ARE:
A. Amphetamines
B. Barbiturates
C. Rauwolfia alkaloids
D. Major antidepressants
E. Major tranquilizers
Ref. 367 - p. 376

866. PREOCCUPATION WITH A SINGLE ACTIVITY WHICH MAY BE CARRIED ON INCESSANTLY IS OFTEN SEEN IN ADDICTS INGESTING LARGE DOSES OF:
A. Heroin
B. Barbiturates
C. Marijuana
D. Amphetamines
E. Alcohol
Ref. 367 - p. 379

867. THE IMPROVEMENT BROUGHT ABOUT BY AMPHETAMINES IN HYPERACTIVE CHILDREN WITH MINIMAL BRAIN DYSFUNCTION (MBD) SYNDROME IS PROBABLY RELATED TO ITS EFFECT ON:
A. REM activity
B. Constituent EEG sleep stages
C. Affect
D. Attention
E. Drowsiness
Ref. 367 - p. 377

131

868. THE PREVALENCE OF PSYCHOTHERAPEUTIC DRUG USE IN A CROSS-
SECTION SAMPLE OF ADULT WOMEN IN SAN FRANCISCO IS:
   A. 5%
   B. 10%
   C. 25%
   D. 33%
   E. 45%   Ref. 367 - p. 385

869. THE PREVALENCE OF PSYCHOTHERAPEUTIC DRUG USE IN A CROSS-
SECTION SAMPLE OF ADULT MEN IN SAN FRANCISCO IS:
   A. 5%
   B. 10%
   C. 25%
   D. 33%
   E. 45%   Ref. 367 - p. 385

870. THE NOSIE IS A:
   A. Computer-based diagnostic method
   B. Device for increasing the safety of ECT
   C. Patient evaluation for nurses
   D. Phenomenon occurring in Capgras' syndrome
   E. A nosology based on DSM-II   Ref. 368 - p. 405

871. THE DURATION OF DRUG-INDUCED EXTRAPYRAMIDAL EFFECTS IS:
   A. So long as the phenothiazine is continued
   B. Lengthened by the use of antiparkinsonism drugs
   C. Unaffected by antiparkinsonism drugs
   D. Often no more than three months
   E. Usually prolonged even after the cessation of phenothiazines
                                     Ref. 369 - p. 411

872. DRUGS WHICH MAY CAUSE NEUROLOGICAL SIDE-EFFECTS SIMILAR TO
AN IDIOPATHIC PARKINSON SYNDROME ARE:
   A. Butyrophenones
   B. Thioxanthenes
   C. Phenothiazines
   D. All of the above
   E. None of the above   Ref. 369 - p. 410

873. OF THE EXTRAPYRAMIDAL REACTIONS INDUCED BY NEUROLEPTIC
DRUGS, THE ONE WHOSE TIME OF ONSET GENERALLY IS WITHIN THE
FIRST 4-1/2 DAYS IS:
   A. Dyskinesia
   B. Rigidity
   C. Tremor
   D. Akinesia
   E. Tardive dyskinesia   Ref. 369 - p. 411

874. PATIENTS WHO RECEIVE NEUROLEPTIC DRUGS SHOULD BE TREATED
WITH CONCOMITANT ANTIPARKINSONIAN MEDICATION BECAUSE:
   A. Antiparkinsonian medications have few if any adverse side effects
   B. Parkinsonian symptoms usually will recur if they are withdrawn
   C. Parkinsonian symptoms are likely to develop at any time during
      anti-psychotic medication therapy
   D. All of the above
   E. None of the above   Ref. 369 - p. 410

875. TIME TENDS TO BE EXPERIENCED AS "SPEEDED UP" WITH:
   A. Sensory deprivation
   B. Sensory overload
   C. Dreaming
   D. Neuroleptic drugs
   E. Solitary confinement   Ref. 370 - p. 413

876. THE CONSTRUCT OF STIMULUS OVERLOAD SEEMS PLAUSIBLE TO
   ACCOUNT FOR THE ALTERATIONS OF CONSCIOUSNESS FOUND IN:
   A. Hypnopompic states
   B. Break-off phenomena in high altitude jet pilots
   C. Hyperkinetic trance states
   D. Nocturnal hallucinations
   E. Postcataract operation psychoses   Ref. 370 - p. 414

877. SENSORY DEPRIVATION APPEARS TO ACCOUNT FOR THE ALTERATIONS
   OF CONSCIOUSNESS FOUND IN:
   A. The "third degree"
   B. Battle fatigue
   C. Revival meetings
   D. Road hypnosis
   E. All of the above   Ref. 370 - p. 414

878. THE COMPULSION TO REPEAT TRAUMATIC EVENTS IS REFLECTED
   IN:
   A. Unbidden images
   B. Obsessive ideas
   C. Nightmares
   D. Recurrent emotional states
   E. All of the above   Ref. 371 - p. 419

879. THE GREAT TRUISM OF INFORMATION THEORY IS:
   A. Information is a product of input and accessibility
   B. Reflected in the operation of the computer-controlled EEG
   C. Found in the behavior of persons subjected to brain washing techniques
   D. A variable cannot be controlled unless information about the variable
      is available to the controller
   E. Information is unavailable to the subject unless it is expressed in terms
      that can be processed   Ref. 372 - p. 436

880. PSYCHOPHYSIOLOGICAL VARIABLES CAN BE CONTROLLED BY THE
   USE OF EXTERNAL FEEDBACK WHEN:
   A. The variable is electronically measured
   B. The variable is made into an output
   C. The variable is fed back to the subject producing it through a sensory
      channel
   D. The variable is made into an input
   E. All of the above   Ref. 372 - p. 436

881. ALPHA RHYTHM CAN BE BROUGHT UNDER VOLUNTARY CONTROL
   THROUGH THE USE OF:
   A. Phecyclidine (Sernyl)
   B. Chlorpromazine
   C. LSD
   D. Processed EEG signals
   E. All of the above   Ref. 372 - p. 436

882. A MAJOR FACTOR DIFFERENTIATING FEEDBACK OF OPERANT CONDITIONING FROM OTHER FEEDBACK IS:
A. The absence of instrumental methods
B. The valence of the feedback
C. Impermanence of the resulting conditioning
D. Inability to predict result
E. None of the above   Ref. 372 - p. 438

883. IN THE CLASSIFICATION OF SIGNALS, THOSE WHICH ARE DISCONTINUOUS ARE DESIGNATED AS:
A. Analog
B. Digital
C. Synthetic
D. Diacritic
E. Anomalous   Ref. 372 - p. 438

884. ALPHA ACTIVITY IS ASSOCIATED IN EEG FEEDBACK SUBJECTS WITH:
A. Tranquil state of mind
B. High state of alertness
C. Restlessness
D. Arousal
E. Suspiciousness   Ref. 372 - p. 439

885. THETA ACTIVITY IS ASSOCIATED IN EEG FEEDBACK SUBJECTS WITH:
A. Pleasure
B. Drowsiness
C. Tranquillity
D. Restlessness
E. Meditative state   Ref. 372 - p. 439

886. THE PREDOMINANT REASON FOR PURSUING THE STUDY OF EMG FEEDBACK IS THE:
A. Use of this method in the treatment of paralysis following cerebrovascular accidents
B. Finding that complete muscle relaxation is incompatible with anxiety
C. Use of EMG activity variations for lie detection purposes
D. Attempt to influence regeneration of muscle following destruction of neural supply
E. Relative economy involved compared to EEG feedback
                                       Ref. 372 - p. 439

887. SO FAR, THE MAJOR THERAPEUTIC USE OF FEEDBACK HAS BEEN IN THE TREATMENT OF:
A. Muscle tension
B. Hypertension
C. Vasoconstrictive peripheral vascular disease
D. Anxiety
E. Epilepsy   Ref. 372 - p. 440

888. EMG FEEDBACK STUDIES HAVE DEMONSTRATED A COMPLETE ABSENCE OF EMG ACTIVITY IN:
A. Frontalis muscle
B. Temporalis muscle
C. Postural muscle
D. All of the above
E. None of the above   Ref. 372 - p. 439

889. THE THEORY THAT EACH FAMILY DEVELOPS ITS OWN DISTINCTIVE
VIEW OF ITS ENVIRONMENT IS KNOWN AS:
A. Family schism
B. Family skew
C. Consensual experience
D. Consensual validation
E. Cognitive dissonance   Ref. 373 - p. 442

890. ENVIRONMENT-SENSITIVE FAMILIES:
A. Experience their environment as disorganized
B. Stick together as a form of mutual protection
C. Form fixed, stylized notions about the environment
D. Tune their cognitive and perceptual sensitivities toward maintaining
consensus
E. Regard the thoughts and actions of others in the family as a rich
source of information about the environment
Ref. 373 - p. 442

891. CONSENSUS-SENSITIVE FAMILIES:
A. Experience each other as the only regular protection from a hostile
environment
B. Have their perceptual and cognitive sensitivity tuned primarily toward
the environment
C. Experience the environment as governed by a set of discoverable
principles
D. Are involved and invested in their environment
E. Have their perceptual and cognitive sensitivity tuned through the
observation of the interaction of other family members with the
environment   Ref. 373 - p. 442

892. AS INTERMEMBER ACCESS IS DIMINISHED, FAMILY PROBLEM SOLVING
ABILITIES ARE:
A. Diminished in consensus-sensitive families
B. Improved in consensus-sensitive families
C. Unchanged in consensus-sensitive families
D. Improved in environment-sensitive families
E. Diminished in environment-sensitive families
Ref. 373 - p. 442

893. AMONG THOSE WHO ATTEMPT SUICIDE:
A. Men outnumber women by 2 to 3:1
B. Women outnumber men by 2 to 3:1
C. Men slightly outnumber women
D. Women slightly outnumber men
E. The proportion of men to women is about 1:1
Ref. 374 - p. 468

894. SUICIDE ATTEMPTS BY WRIST CUTTING:
A. Usually occur in those over 30
B. Rarely occur in men
C. Are seen more often in married persons
D. All of the above
E. None of the above   Ref. 374 - p. 468

895. ACCORDING TO THOMAS SZASZ, THE USE OF ADDICTING DRUGS:
      A. Must be controlled by stricter laws
      B. Frequently leads to heightened creativity
      C. Is a right of the individual
      D. Is a result of a permissive society
      E. Should be prohibited except when prescribed by a psychiatrist for the
          treatment of a more serious addiction
                                              Ref. 375 - p. 546

896. THE AIM OF SZASZ'S POSITION APPEARS TO BE:
      A. Improvement of the hospital treatment of drug addiction
      B. Having addicts treated in the office rather than in a hospital setting
      C. Increased use of methadone in the treatment of addiction
      D. Restriction of heroin use to confirmed addicts
      E. Forcing us to re-examine our established views
                                              Ref. 376 - p. 548

897. SZASZ MAKES A CALL FOR INCREASED:
      A. Research
      B. Delivery of available medical facilities
      C. Use of methadone
      D. Government funding
      E. Personal responsibility   Ref. 376 - p. 548

898. THE MOST FAVORABLE TREATMENT PROSPECTS ARE FOUND IN
      THOSE MEMBERS OF THE HEROIN COPPING COMMUNITY WHO ARE:
      A. Workers
      B. Big dealers
      C. Street dealers
      D. Bag followers
      E. Touts   Ref. 377 - p. 555

899. IN THE HEROIN COPPING COMMUNITY, THOSE WHO HAVE BEEN
      ADDICTS THE LONGEST ARE THE:
      A. Hustlers
      B. Bag followers
      C. Touts
      D. Workers
      E. Dealers   Ref. 377 - p. 553

900. THE AVERAGE WEEKLY COST OF A HEROIN HABIT IS:
      A. $ 10
      B. $ 50
      C. $ 100
      D. $ 200
      E. $ 500   Ref. 377 - p. 553

901. THE USE OF THE MMPI IN AUTOMATED MULTIPHASIC HEALTH TESTING
      (AMHT):
      A. Is suitable for the general screening of previously unselected populations
      B. Has a high degree of patient acceptance
      C. Is feasible because it was developed as a screening instrument
      D. Is not suitable since many persons resent having to answer many highly
          personal questions
      E. Is suitable because it is primarily a diagnostic tool for those already
          identified as emotionally distressed   Ref. 378 - p. 561

902. AN INDICATOR WHICH HAS BEEN SHOWN TO BE RELATED TO EMOTIO-
NAL STATE AND CORONARY HEART DISEASE IS:
A. Finger-print pattern
B. Voice pattern
C. Eye color
D. Hair length
E. Hair color   Ref. 378 - p. 562

903. A BLOOD TEST WHICH HAS BEEN SHOWN TO BE RELATED TO ACHIEVE-
MENT AND ACHIEVEMENT-ORIENTED BEHAVIOR IS:
A. Uric acid
B. BUN
C. VDRL
D. FBS
E. Etiocholanolone   Ref. 378 - p. 562

904. A STRONG RELATIONSHIP HAS BEEN FOUND BETWEEN EMOTIONAL
DISTRESS AND SERUM:
A. Cholesterol
B. Albumin
C. Potassium
D. Sodium
E. Amylase   Ref. 378 - p. 562

905. THE PSYCHIATRIC SCREENING INSTRUMENT BEST SUITED FOR
AUTOMATED MULTIPHASIC HEALTH TESTING IS:
A. Verbal part of the WAIS
B. Figure drawing
C. MMPI
D. Set of questions related to patients' psychiatric symptoms that is
highly correlated with psychiatric impairment
E. Free-association interview   Ref. 378 - p. 561

906. THE SPHERE WHICH IS DISTURBED IN MANIA IS:
A. Affectivity
B. Attention
C. Perception
D. Language
E. All of the above   Ref. 379 - p. 564

907. A DRUG WHICH IS REPORTED TO INFLUENCE VERBAL LEARNING IS:
A. L-dopa
B. L-tryptophan
C. Propranol
D. All of the above
E. None of the above   Ref. 379 - p. 565

908. THE HIGHEST PROPORTION OF IDIOSYNCRATIC ASSOCIATION RE-
SPONSES OCCURS IN:
A. Psychotic depressives
B. Manics
C. Schizophrenia
D. Psychoses induced by DOM
E. Psychoses induced by DOET   Ref. 379 - p. 572

909. AROUSAL INFLUENCES LEARNING:
      A. When it is at maximal levels
      B. When it is at minimal levels
      C. According to an inverted-U function
      D. In a straight line gradient
      E. In reciprocal terms   Ref. 379 - p. 571

910. DISTURBANCE OF THE LONGER-TERM LEARNING FUNCTIONS OF
      RECENT MEMORY IS ASSOCIATED WITH:
      A. Psychotic depression
      B. Mania
      C. Schizophrenia
      D. All of the above
      E. None of the above   Ref. 379 - p. 572

911. THE LONGER-TERM LEARNING FUNCTION OF RECENT MEMORY
      INVOLVES:
      A. Encoding and organizing bits of information
      B. Transferring bits of information back and forth to storage systems
      C. Retaining bits of information in storage for a short time
      D. Retrieving bits of information from storage
      E. All of the above   Ref. 379 - p. 568

912. A USEFUL INDICATOR OF SEXUAL AROUSAL IN THE MALE IS:
      A. Urinary acid phosphatase
      B. Urinary transaminase
      C. SGOT
      D. LDH
      E. LH   Ref. 380 - p. 580

913. EXPERIMENTAL DATA SUPPORT THE HYPOTHESIS THAT REPEATED
      EXPOSURE TO PORNOGRAPHY RESULTS IN:
      A. Paranoid trends
      B. Decreased responsiveness to it
      C. Homosexual preoccupation
      D. Castration anxiety
      E. Acting out   Ref. 380 - p. 581

914. REPEATED ALLUSION TO AN ADOPTED CHILD'S ADOPTION:
      A. Is necessary for the development in the child of a sense of basic trust
      B. Conveys a sense of trust and respect for the integrity of the child
      C. Is desirable since the child usually discovers this at some point from
          others
      D. All of the above
      E. None of the above   Ref. 381 - p. 591

915. ADOPTION AGENCIES USUALLY:
      A. Withhold any information regarding the biological parents
      B. Caution against telling the child it is adopted
      C. Are not sought out by the adoptive parents when they are troubled about
          their child
      D. All of the above
      E. None of the above   Ref. 381 - p. 592

138

916. COLLABORATION BETWEEN MENTAL HEALTH FACILITIES AND
ADOPTION AGENCIES IS AN EXAMPLE OF:
A. Primary prevention
B. Secondary prevention
C. Tertiary prevention
D. All of the above
E. None of the above   Ref. 381 - p. 590

917. THE LANGNER PSYCHIATRIC IMPAIRMENT SCALE DETECTS:
A. Organic brain syndromes
B. Mental retardation
C. Sociopathic disorders
D. All of the above
E. None of the above   Ref. 382 - p. 601

918. THE GREATEST VALUE OF THE LANGNER PSYCHIATRIC IMPAIRMENT
SCALE APPEARS TO BE IN:
A. The detection of neurotics
B. Assessing the individual
C. Those who externalize and project their emotional problems
D. Those who use denial
E. Marked psychoses   Ref. 382 - p. 601

IN QUESTIONS 919 - 1080 CHOOSE:

A. If only 1, 2, and 3 are correct
B. If only 1 and 3 are correct
C. If only 2 and 4 are correct
D. If only 4 is correct
E. If all are correct

919. DIAGNOSIS OF HYSTERICAL FITS RESTS ON THE FINDING OF:
1. Flexor plantar reflexes
2. Absence of tongue-biting
3. Absence of bed-wetting or incontinence
4. Rigidity of the muscles   Ref. 383 - p. 603

920. THE TREATMENT OF HYSTERICAL FITS BY PAINFUL ELECTRIC
SHOCKS:
1. Utilizes "punishment"
2. Is an example of classical conditioning
3. Is an example of operant conditioning
4. Involves induction of a seizure   Ref. 383 - p. 602

921. MANIFESTATION OF HYSTERIA SUCH AS FITS, TRANCES, AND
PARALYSIS:
1. Are still encountered frequently in clinical practice in the U.S.A.
2. Probably occur in those with underlying organic disorders
3. Are not amenable to psychological treatment
4. Are frequently encountered in clinical practice in India
                                      Ref. 383 - p. 602

922. ON THE THIRD DAY OF PHENOTHIAZINE TREATMENT THERE IS A
DECREASE IN:
1. Drowsiness
2. Dryness of the mouth
3. Postural hypotension
4. Parkinsonism   Ref. 384 - p. 641

923. THE STACCATO SYNDROME:
1. Occurs in patients on phenothiazines having parkinsonian side effects
2. Is complicated by multiple drug abuse
3. Is best treated with antiparkinsonian drugs
4. Is helped by a short period of phenothiazine medication
                                   Ref. 385 - p. 647

924. MANIC PATIENTS CAN BE DIVIDED INTO SUBGROUPS CHARACTERIZED
AS:
1. Submissive-passive
2. Elated-grandiose
3. Congenial-altruistic
4. Paranoid-destructive   Ref. 386 - p. 693

925. SYMPTOMS FREQUENTLY FOUND IN MANIC PATIENTS INCLUDE:
1. Poor judgment
2. Hyperactivity
3. Diminished impulse control
4. Depression   Ref. 386 - p. 689

926. CORE CHARACTERISTICS OF MANIA FOUND IN ALL SUBGROUPS
INCLUDE:
1. Poor judgment
2. Increased social contact
3. Anger
4. Euphoria   Ref. 386 - p. 693

927. THE NATIVE AMERICAN CHURCH OF NORTH AMERICA:
1. Practices polygamy
2. Advocates strict abstinence from alcohol
3. Is composed of only one Indian tribe
4. Uses a hallucinogen in religious ceremonies
                                   Ref. 387 - p. 695

928. AMONG THE PSYCHOPHARMACOLOGICALLY SIGNIFICANT ALKALOIDS
IN PEYOTE IS:
1. Ergotamine
2. Papaverine
3. Cannabis
4. Mescaline   Ref. 387 - p. 695

929. HARMFUL SIDE EFFECTS OF PEYOTE ARE MINIMIZED IN THE
AMERICAN INDIAN CHURCH WHICH USES IT BY:
1. Emphasis on the real world rather than introspection
2. Emphasis on adherence to societal standards rather than freeing of
impulses
3. Positive expectation
4. Availability of chlorpromazine Ref. 387 - p. 697

930. DIABETIC PATIENTS CHARACTERISTICALLY RESPOND TO STRESS BY:
 1. Withdrawal
 2. Development of insulin tolerance
 3. Increased use of insulin
 4. Overeating   Ref. 388 - p. 700

931. DEVELOPMENT OF AN ULCER IN AN INDIVIDUAL APPEARS TO BE A
 FUNCTION OF:
 1. High pepsinogen secretion
 2. Sensitivity to beef protein
 3. Unresolved conflicts about oral gratification and dependency
 4. Unresolved oedipal guilt   Ref. 388 - p. 700

932. IN THE STUDY OF JUVENILE DIABETICS THERE IS A FINDING OF:
 1. High incidence of loss
 2. Significant number of one-parent families
 3. Severe family disturbance
 4. Relatively high socioeconomic position of family
                                        Ref. 388 - p. 703

933. DURING THE PREMENSTRUAL AND MENSTRUAL PHASE OF THE CYCLE
 THERE IS AN INCREASED INCIDENCE OF:
 1. Suicide attempts
 2. Relapse in manic patients
 3. Relapse in schizophrenic patients
 4. Hospitalization for depression   Ref. 389 - p. 705

934. FEWER PREMENSTRUAL SUICIDE ATTEMPTS ARE MADE IN WOMEN
 WHO:
 1. Complain of premenstrual symptoms
 2. Do not complain of premenstrual symptoms
 3. Are not living with a male partner
 4. Are living with a male partner   Ref. 389 - p. 709

935. WOMEN WITH A HISTORY OF MEDICAL AND SEXUAL PROBLEMS ARE
 MORE LIKELY TO MANIFEST DURING THE WEEK PRECEDING
 MENSTRUATION:
 1. Hostility
 2. Suicidal ideation
 3. Suicide attempts
 4. Feelings of well-being   Ref. 389 - p. 709

936. THE "MAMA'S BOY" SYNDROME OCCURS IN CHILDREN:
 1. Who are usually referred for counseling during the pre-school years
 2. Who are good achievers
 3. Whose mothers are overly punitive
 4. Who are frequently called "sissy" or "baby" by peers
                                        Ref. 390 - p. 712

937. CHILDREN WITH THE "MAMA'S BOY" SYNDROME:
 1. Usually make a satisfactory adjustment after psychotherapy
 2. Have overprotective mothers who infantilize them
 3. Usually benefit from psychotropic medication
 4. Benefit from short-term hospitalization
                                        Ref. 390 - p. 712

938. HOSPITALIZATION OF THE CHILD WITH SYMBIOTIC PSYCHOSIS:
1. Brings about further growth
2. Leads to improved social relations
3. Is useful when the mother cannot cooperate in family treatment
4. May result in further withdrawal and deterioration
                                        Ref. 390 - p. 716

939. MOTIVATION FOR PSYCHOTHERAPY:
1. Implies a desire for change
2. Implies a desire for relief of symptoms
3. Is a crucial selection criterion for psychotherapy
4. Has little prognostic significance   Ref. 391 - p. 719

940. HELMHOLTZ:
1. Published a study of physiognomy
2. Developed the ophthalmoscope
3. Wrote the classic nineteenth century German textbook of psychiatry
4. Showed the connection between the nerve cell and nerve fiber
                                        Ref. 392 - p. 731

941. PINEL:
1. Was superintendent of the Bicetre
2. Was superintendent of the Salpetriere
3. Introduced humanitarian methods in the treatment of the mentally ill
4. Used moral treatment   Ref. 392 - p. 729

942. WALTER CANNON:
1. Discovered sympathin, produced by the adrenal medulla
2. Wrote "Bodily Changes in Pain, Hunger, Fear and Rage"
3. Developed the concept of homeostasis
4. Studies dreams   Ref. 392 - p. 733

943. A PSYCHOSIS IN ONE PARTNER IN A MARRIAGE:
1. Is often reported as leading to growing mutual understanding
2. Is often best treated by activity involving the nonpsychotic spouse
   in the treatment process
3. Can be effectively dealt with as a marital crisis
4. Is generally the result of a disturbance in the marriage
                                        Ref. 393 - p. 735

944. WOMEN WHO HAVE UNWANTED PREGNANCIES TEND TO:
1. Have excessive dependency needs
2. Have unresolved passive-agressive conflicts
3. Be ambivalent toward men
4. Use the mechanism of denial   Ref. 394 - p. 743

945. THE BIRTH RATE AMONG HOSPITALIZED AND FORMERLY HOSPITAL-
IZED MENTALLY ILL WOMEN:
1. Appears to be increasing due to partial hospitalization and day care
2. Appears to be increasing due to rapid discharge
3. Appears to be increasing due to drug maintenance in the community
4. Appears to be decreasing   Ref. 394 - p. 743

946. THE PSYCHOLOGICAL ORGANIZATION OF THE HYSTERICAL PERSONAL-
ITY IS CHARACTERIZED BY A COGNITIVE STYLE WHICH IS:
1. Impressionistic
2. Global
3. Immediate
4. Conducive to ego disruption   Ref. 395 - p. 745

947. HYSTERICAL PSYCHOSIS:
1. Seldom lasts longer than one to three weeks
2. Has clinical manifestations which include hallucinations and delusions
3. Occurs in hysterical personalities
4. Often leaves a residual defect   Ref. 395 - p. 745

948. TYPES OF HYSTERICAL PSYCHOSIS CAN RESULT FROM THE PROCESS
OF:
1. Culturally sanctioned behavior
2. Appropriation of psychotic behavior as the expression of a conversion
symptom involving a reinforcement of repression
3. Disruption and breakdown of ego boundaries involving a failure of
repression
4. Fragmentation of thinking   Ref. 395 - p. 745

949. THE MARRIAGES OF WOMEN WHO DEVELOP A HYSTERICAL PSYCHOSIS
TEND TO BE:
1. Based on a bond of hatred
2. Characterized by chronic moderate crises
3. Characterized by acute severe crises
4. Symbiotic   Ref. 395 - p. 748

950. IN THE EXPLORATORY TIME-LIMITED CONSULTATIVE PROCESS IN
WOMEN WITH UNWANTED PREGNANCIES, THERE IS THERAPEUTIC
VALUE IN THE PATIENT'S DEVELOPING AWARENESS OF:
1. Acting out
2. Narcissism
3. The need to be pregnant
4. Life-long depressive practices   Ref. 396 - p. 751

951. MOTHERHOOD IN TEEN-AGE GIRLS PRESENTS A PROBLEM IN THAT:
1. It may predispose to increased weight gain
2. It may predispose to toxemia
3. Self-defeating cycles of further pregnancies occur
4. They may drop out of school   Ref. 397 - p. 758

952. IN THE METROPOLITAN HOSPITAL STUDY OF TEEN-AGE MOTHERS,
MOST OF THE GIRLS:
1. Come from broken homes without a father
2. Are married at the time of delivery
3. Were amenable to treatment in a group setting
4. Expressed guilt and shame   Ref. 397 - p. 759

953. SIGNIFICANT ELEMENTS OF SUPPORTIVE PSYCHOTHERAPY INCLUDE:
1. Expressions of interest and solicitude
2. Giving advice
3. Ventilation
4. Interpretation of transference   Ref. 398 - p. 763

954. A PSYCHIATRIC TRIAGE UNIT:
1. Emphasizes long-term treatment
2. Deals with primary and tertiary prevention
3. Avoids the use of psychotropic medication
4. Employs a sorting process as part of the evaluation and treatment
   program   Ref. 399 - p. 771

955. IN A PSYCHIATRIC TRIAGE PROGRAM IT IS IMPORTANT THAT:
1. The unit be located in the midst of the patient catchment area
2. The ward environment not be comfortable
3. Neighborhood workers and volunteers be used
4. There be an exposure of small numbers of patients to relatively
   large numbers of professional staff
                                             Ref. 399 - p. 772

956. A RECENT STUDY FROM ENGLAND HAS FOUND THAT ASSOCIATED
WITH CONSISTENT CANNABIS SMOKING OVER A PERIOD OF THREE TO
ELEVEN YEARS HAS BEEN NOTED:
1. Significant cerebral atrophy
2. Grand mal seizures
3. Damage in the region of the caudate nuclei, basal ganglia and
   structures adjacent to the third ventricle
4. Hypertensive encephalopathy   Ref. 400 - p. 1223

957. WOLPE'S TECHNIQUE OF SYSTEMATIC DESENSITIZATION EMPLOYS
A STRATEGY OF:
1. Tachistoscopic induction of dream content
2. Fantasy induction
3. Fantasy interpretation
4. Deep muscle relaxation   Ref. 401 - p. 7

958. IN PRIMARY ANOREXIA NERVOSA THE PATHOGNOMIC FEATURE IS:
1. Dramatic denial of illness
2. Absence of concern over advanced emaciation
3. Stubborn defense of an often gruesome appearance
4. Complaint about weight loss   Ref. 402 - p. 52

959. IN THE BACKGROUND OF PRIMARY ANOREXIA NERVOSA PATIENTS:
1. The parents have been uninvolved and withholding of advantages and
   privileges
2. There is a disregard of child-initiated signals
3. There is a minimal stress on success, outer appearances and beauty
4. The oppositional phase of early childhood is characteristically absent
                                             Ref. 402 - p. 52

960. THE PSYCHOTHERAPEUTIC APPROACH IN PRIMARY ANOREXIA
NERVOSA SHOULD PLACE EMPHASIS ON:
1. Interpretation of oral aggression
2. Investigation of the function of eating in the life of the patient
3. Exhortation to eat
4. Evoking awareness of feelings and impulses that originate in the
   patients themselves   Ref. 402 - p. 51

144

961. A MODIFICATION OF PARANOID SYMPTOMS BY PLACEBO TREATMENT
TAKES PLACE IN PARANOID PATIENTS WHO:
1. Have a positive response propensity
2. Have a negative response propensity
3. Are socially isolated, non-belligerent and cognitively undifferentiated
4. Are socially involved, belligerent and cognitively differentiated
Ref. 403 - p. 68

962. INDIVIDUALS WHO PERFORM IN A FIELD-DEPENDENT MANNER:
1. Have a poor sense of separate identity
2. Use massive repression and primitive denial
3. Have a diffuse and global body concept
4. Rarely have problems with alcohol   Ref. 404 - p. 77

963. PSYCHOTROPIC AGENTS PRODUCING PSYCHOMOTOR RETARDATION
AND SEDATION, CAUSE MARKED DISCOMFORT IN:
1. Manifestly passive individuals
2. Anxious persons
3. Introverted individuals
4. Extroverted athletes   Ref. 405 - p. 92

964. COMPARED TO THERAPISTS WITH A HIGH DROP-OUT RATE
THERAPISTS WITH A LOW DROP-OUT RATE FOR LOW CLASS PATIENTS
ON DRUG TREATMENT:
1. Rate their patients higher in pathology
2. Rate their patients with a better prognosis
3. Report greater liking for their patients
4. Are more active   Ref. 406 - p. 103

965. 2, 5-DIMETHOXY-4-METHYLAMPHETAMINE (DOM):
1. Produces LSD-like symptoms
2. Is found in samples of STP
3. Causes significant increases in anxiety
4. Raises blood pressure and pulse rate markedly
Ref. 407 - p. 119

966. FAMILIAL AND NON-FAMILIAL SCHIZOPHRENICS HAVE BEEN REPORTED
BY MARICQ TO HAVE DIFFERENCES IN:
1. Hair color
2. Pupillary shape
3. Head shape
4. Visibility of nailfold capillary plexus
Ref. 408 - p. 146

967. VERBALLY INDUCED BEHAVIORAL RESPONSES DURING SLEEP:
1. Cannot occur without significant change in alpha frequency
2. Occur mainly in stages 3 and 4
3. Are repeated by the subject following similar cues when awake
4. Are not remembered by the subjects when awake
Ref. 409 - p. 171

968. COMPARED TO REM SLEEP AWAKENINGS FOLLOWING AWAKENING
FROM NON-REM SLEEP, REPORTS OF PRE-AWAKENING EXPERIENCES
TEND TO BE:
1. Longer
2. Less bizarre
3. More emotional
4. More thoughtlike   Ref. 410 - p. 188

969. COMPARED TO RESPONSES AFTER SLEEP, RESPONSES TO THE TAT
AFTER AWAKENING FROM NON-REM SLEEP ARE:
1. Less bizarre
2. Less emotional
3. Less imaginative
4. Less negative in affective tone   Ref. 410 - p. 189

970. WHEN THE VISUAL STIMULUS WAS FLASHED BEFORE THE SUBJECTS
RETIRED TO BED, FREE ASSOCIATION RESPONSES ON THE REBUS
LEVEL WERE OBTAINED FOLLOWING:
1. Stage 3
2. Stage 4
3. Stage 2
4. REM stage   Ref. 411 - p. 196

971. THE SUBJECT'S OWN VOICE, PRESENTED TO THE SUBJECT DURING
HIS SLEEP, RESULTS IN DREAMS:
1. In which the dreamer is in a passive position
2. Which are more colorful and bizarre
3. Which have a frightening content
4. In which the dreamer is represented as active and assertive
                                      Ref. 411 - p. 196

972. AS COMPARED TO REM SLEEP, THERE IS IN STAGE 2 SLEEP A
LIKELIHOOD OF:
1. Reality-attuned thinking
2. Problem solving
3. Learning
4. More pleasant mental experience   Ref. 411 - p. 200

973. COMPARED TO STAGE 1 REM, STAGE 2:
1. Imagery is more unclear
2. Imagery is more ambiguous
3. Thinking is more realistic
4. Thinking is more secondary process in nature
                                      Ref. 411 - p. 200

974. THE PICTURES PAINTED BY DEPRESSIVES CONTAIN THE FOLLOWING
ELEMENTS:
1. Upper portion darkest
2. Immobile figures
3. Trees broken off and no flowers
4. Starless nights rather than days   Ref. 411 - p. 216

975. PAINTING DONE DURING A MANIC PERIOD TENDS TO HAVE:
1. Vivid colors
2. Bold lines
3. Loose organization
4. Only a part of the field is filled   Ref. 412 - p. 222

976. COMPARED TO NON-ARTISTS, ARTISTS MANIFEST ON THE RORSCHACH:
1. High degree of originality in perception
2. Diminished ease of regression
3. High degree of diffuse anxiety
4. Fixity of ego boundaries   Ref. 413 - p. 241

977. THE RORSCHACH RECORDS OF ARTISTS CONTAIN:
1. High numbers of human movement responses
2. Many color responses
3. Large numbers of whole responses
4. Good form level   Ref. 413 - p. 234

978. POSSIBLE TARGETS FOR USE IN THE PSYCHOSURGICAL TREATMENT
OF THE PATIENT WITH INTRACTABLE DEPRESSION INCLUDE:
1. Posterior medial frontal area
2. Congulum
3. Dorsal medial nucleus
4. Anterior nucleus of the thalamus   Ref. 414 - p. 266

979. THE DANGER OF SUICIDE IN THE DEPRESSED PATIENT IS MOST
ACCENTUATED DURING THE PERIOD:
1. Of psychomotor retardation
2. Preceding the peak of the depression
3. Of the peak of the depression
4. Following the peak of the depression Ref. 414 - p. 272

980. THE TREATMENT OF PSYCHOMOTOR EPILEPSY BY STEREOTACTIC
IMPLANTATION OF DEPTH ELECTRODES, COMPARED TO TEMPORAL
LOBECTOMY IS:
1. Less hazardous
2. Followed by less decrement on psychometric measurements
3. Less successful in providing seizure relief
4. Not destructive of brain tissue   Ref. 415 - p. 273

981. PROMINENT IN PATIENTS SURGICALLY TREATED FOR TEMPORAL
LOBE EPILEPSY IS:
1. Identity disturbance associated with the necessity to acquire a
non-epileptic identity
2. Paranoia
3. Depression
4. Mania   Ref. 415 - p. 287

982. SELF-MUTILATION IN SCHIZOPHRENIC CHILDREN IS RELATED TO:
1. Treatment with LSD
2. Physical abuse by the parents during the first 2 years of life
3. Other people being physically present
4. Atmosphere of rejection and stimulus deprivation
        Ref. 416 - p. 373

983.	DURING THE FIRST THREE MONTHS OF LIFE RAPID EYE MOVEMENTS
MAY OCCUR WHEN:
1.	There is sucking
2.	There is fussing
3.	There is crying
4.	Eyes are open			Ref. 417 - p. 377

984.	AT AGE THREE MONTHS THERE IS A MAJOR CHANGE IN REM IN THAT:
1.	Differentiated REM disappears
2.	Undifferentiated REM disappears
3.	The sleep cycle begins with REM
4.	The sleep cycle begins with NREM	Ref. 417 - p. 776

985.	ABRUPT WITHDRAWAL OF NEUROLEPTIC DRUGS MAY LEAD TO:
1.	Nausea and vomiting
2.	Vertigo
3.	Tachycardia
4.	Intensification of parkinsonian side effects
					Ref. 418 - p. 400

986.	IN THE FAMILY CONSTELLATION OF ALCOHOLICS, IT IS FREQUENTLY
FOUND THAT:
1.	Mothers overtly seduce and manipulate their children
2.	There are usually two other siblings or more
3.	There is an absence of a warm, giving relationship with a mother
figure during the early years of development
4.	The alcoholic is the family member who is most ill
					Ref. 419 - p. 430

987.	IN THE PSYCHOTHERAPY OF ALCOHOLIC PATIENTS IT HAS BEEN
FOUND USEFUL TO:
1.	Attack those defenses which are in the form of character traits
2.	Permit the patient to borrow the therapist's ego and superego
3.	Interdict the use of all alcoholic beverages
4.	Point out the reality of the parents' abnormalities
					Ref. 419 - p. 431

988.	IN THE BACKGROUND OF THE IMPOSTER:
1.	There is a strong father with whom the patient identifies
2.	The relationship with the mother is distant and uninvolved
3.	There is an intense parental relationship which excludes the children
4.	The relationship with the mother is intense and ambivalent and
excludes other relationships	Ref. 420 - p. 447

989.	AS OPPOSED TO BILATERAL ECT, UNILATERAL ECT IS ASSOCIATED
WITH:
1.	Less memory impairment and confusion
2.	Diminished clinical effectiveness two to three months later
3.	More symptoms immediately after treatment
4.	Petit mal seizures			Ref. 421 - p. 487

990. A HISTORY OF PREGNANCY AND BIRTH COMPLICATIONS IS OFTEN
FOUND IN THE HISTORIES OF:
1. Depressives
2. Schizophrenics
3. Neurotics
4. Children with behavior disorders   Ref. 422 - p. 24

991. IN SOME WOMEN, ORAL CONTRACEPTIVES LEAD TO THE ADVERSE
PSYCHOLOGICAL REACTION OF:
1. Depressive reactions
2. Lethargy
3. Diminished libido
4. Increased sexual interest   Ref. 423 - p. 40

992. FOLLOW-UP QUESTIONNAIRES REVEAL THAT UNDER THE CALIFORNIA
THERAPEUTIC ABORTION LAW, WOMEN GRANTED AN ABORTION FOR
PSYCHIATRIC INDICATIONS REPORT:
1. Serious psychiatric sequelae
2. Prolonged guilt feelings
3. Paranoid response to the physician
4. Decrease in depressive phenomena between two weeks and four months
postoperatively   Ref. 424 - p. 51

993. AMONG THE RELATIVES OF BIPOLAR PATIENTS, COMPARED WITH
THE RELATIVES OF UNIPOLAR PATIENTS:
1. All forms of affective disorder are more common
2. Mania is more frequent
3. The disorder appears sex-linked
4. ECT is more effective   Ref. 425 - p. 61

994. POSTPARTUM PSYCHOSES IN PATIENTS WITH MANIC-DEPRESSIVE
DISEASE:
1. Seem to predispose patients to further postpartum episodes
2. Occur in 50% of the patients
3. Usually occur within the two months following parturition
4. Are more frequent than nonpuerperal episodes during the period at risk
Ref. 425 - p. 60

995. FIELD-DEPENDENT SUBJECTS, WHEN COMPARED WITH FIELD-
INDEPENDENT SUBJECTS:
1. More readily feel guilt as patients in psychotherapy
2. More readily feel shame as patients in psychotherapy
3. Discriminate better on a physiological level
4. Have a higher level of galvanic skin response activity at rest
Ref. 426 - p. 98

996. THE VIEW THAT CHILDREN WHO ARE PSYCHOTIC POSSESS PRIMARY
ORGANIC DISTURBANCES OF THE CNS IS SUPPORTED BY:
1. The finding of lower birth weight in the member of monozygotic twin
pair discordant for schzophrenia
2. The finding that the schizophrenic twins were the ones who almost
always exhibited evidence of CNS dysfunction
3. Bender's finding of atypical plasticity
4. The process-reactive dichotomy viewpoint
Ref. 427 - p. 111

997. DEPRESSED PATIENTS TREATED WITH IMIPRAMINE OR ECT SHOW:
1. A shift to increased calcium retention
2. Decrease in the negative calcium balance
3. Increase in the positive calcium balance
4. Decrease in serum calcium concentration
Ref. 428 - p. 127

998. THERE IS A DECREASE IN TOTAL REM PERIOD TIME:
1. On first nights in the laboratory
2. After hypnotic suggestion
3. Brought about by thirst
4. Following the viewing of a stressful film
Ref. 429 - p. 143

999. IN ELECTROSLEEP TREATMENT, THE PATIENTS:
1. Often feel great discomfort
2. Occasionally develop prolonged apnea
3. Are rendered unconscious during the treatment
4. Do not necessarily sleep during the treatment
Ref. 430 - p. 146

1000. ELECTROSLEEP TREATMENT APPEARS TO BE HELPFUL IN:
1. Schizophrenia
2. Anxiety
3. Psychotic depression
4. Insomnia
Ref. 430 - p. 150

1001. EMPATHY:
1. Involves understanding what another person is feeling from what he says and does
2. Requires sympathy for the other person
3. Is found in infants
4. Cannot be measured
Ref. 431 - p. 169

1002. RECENT STUDIES HAVE DESCRIBED A DEPRESSIVE REACTION IN SCHIZOPHRENIA:
1. When psychotherapy is initiated
2. Following cessation of phenothiazines
3. With the use of day hospitalization as opposed to full-time hospitalization
4. Following remission of psychotic symptomatology
Ref. 432 - p. 203

1003. THE DISTURBANCE OF AFFECT IN SCHIZOPHRENIA IS CHARACTERIZED BY:
1. Rapidity of changing moods
2. Emptiness
3. Impoverishment
4. Deeply felt affect
Ref. 432 - p. 209

1004. IN THE DOG THERE IS A CONSISTENT INCREASE IN HEART RATE IN RESPONSE TO:
1. Other dogs
2. A person entering the room
3. Fear
4. Being petted
Ref. 433 - p. 233

1005. THE DEVELOPMENT OF SOCIAL ATTACHMENTS IN PUPPIES:
1. Is based upon feeding
2. Is deterred by punishment
3. Has no critical period
4. Becomes difficult with totally new objects after 12 weeks of age
Ref. 433 - p. 239

1006. MONKEYS REARED WITH INANIMATE TERRY-CLOTH SURROGATE MOTHERS:
1. Prefer a wire-mother with nursing bottle when available
2. Experience a reciprocity between themselves and the surrogate
3. Show no destructive influence from the experience
4. Manifest behavioral disturbances   Ref. 433 - p. 241

1007. ACCORDING TO RECENT REPORTS, THE BETA ADRENERGIC BLOCKER, PROPRANOLOL:
1. Reduces the intensity of physiological symptoms of anxiety
2. Exerts its anxiolytic effect by its action on neural receptors in the brain
3. Slows the heart rate
4. Stimulates catecholamine-induced liberation of fat from adipose tissue   Ref. 434 - p. 266

1008. THE EFFECT OF CHRONIC ADMINISTRATION OF LITHIUM ON THE EEG INCLUDES:
1. Diffuse slowing
2. Accentuation of focal abnormality
3. Alteration of alpha activity
4. Abolition of average evoked response
Ref. 435 - p. 273

1009. THE EFFECT OF LITHIUM ON THE METABOLISM OF MONOAMINES IN THE RAT BRAIN IS:
1. Decrease in level of deaminized catechol amines
2. Increase in level of deaminized catechol amines
3. Increased norepinephrine
4. Decreased norepinephrine   Ref. 435 - p. 286

1010   AN ESSENTIAL FACTOR IN THE BACKGROUND OF MALE TRANS-SEXUALS IS:
1. Symbiosis with the mother
2. Bisexual depressed mother
3. Psychologically absent father
4. Sibling rivalry   Ref. 436 - p. 295

1011. HIGH FACILITATIVE THERAPISTS TEND TO BE RATED SIGNIFICANTLY HIGHER ON:
1. Frequency of confrontation
2. Positive regard
3. Empathy
4. Concreteness   Ref. 437 - p. 304

1012.   THE TYPES OF CONFRONTATIONS THAT ARE MORE OFTEN OFFERED
        BY HIGH FACILITATIVE THERAPISTS ARE:
        1. Experiential
        2. Didactic
        3. Encouragement to action
        4. Weakness   Ref. 437 - p. 305

1013.   FOLLOWING PSYCHOTHERAPY, AN IMPROVEMENT IN IQ IS CORRE-
        LATED WITH A CHANGE FOR THE BETTER IN:
        1. Self-concept
        2. Ego strength
        3. Patterning of defenses
        4. Symptoms   Ref. 438 - p. 312

1014.   THERE APPEARS TO BE A DISORDER IN SCHIZOPHRENIC CHILDREN:
        1. In the development of lateral preference
        2. Of body image
        3. Of right-left awareness
        4. Discrepancy between mental age and spatial competence
                                          Ref. 439 - p. 350

1015.   THE PATTERNS OF EPIDERMAL RIDGES ON THE VOLAR SURFACES
        OF THE HANDS AND FEET (DERMATOGLYPHICS) ARE:
        1. Largely under genetic control
        2. Abnormal in children suffering from prenatal rubella syndrome
        3. Abnormal in normal children whose mothers were exposed
            to rubella in the first trimester
        4. Formed by the eighteenth fetal week
                                          Ref. 440 - p. 352

1016.   A COMPARISON OF THE ASSESSMENT OF THE DURATION AND TEM-
        PORAL PATTERNING OF SLEEP BY MEANS OF ALL- NIGHT EEG
        RECORDING AND BY SYSTEMATIC NURSING OBSERVATION REVEALS:
        1. Low nursing reliability in assessment of sleep of schizophrenic
            patients
        2. Low nursing reliability in assessment of sleep of depressed patients
        3. No discrepancy in observational reliability between schizophrenic
            and depressed groups
        4. Nursing observation is not a satisfactory method for quantifying
            sleep in depressed patients   Ref. 441 - p. 367

1017.   SLEEP SPEECH (SOMNILOQUY):
        1. Is most frequent during the early part of sleep
        2. Is most frequent prior to awakening
        3. Is most frequent during the latter part of sleep
        4. Is generally associated with NREM sleep rather than REM sleep
                                          Ref. 442 - p. 373

1018.   SLEEP UTTERANCES (VOCALIZATION IN ASSOCIATION WITH SLEEP):
        1. Include laughter and weeping
        2. Are uncommon
        3. Are usually beyond awareness or not remembered
        4. Are not clearly enunciated words   Ref. 442 - p. 369

152

1019. CONCORDANCE BETWEEN THE CONTENT OF SLEEP TALKING AND
MENTATION RECALLED UPON AWAKENING:
1. Is absent in NREM sleep speech
2. Cannot be established on the basis of psychoanalytic interpretation
3. Is only at the level of third order concordance
4. Is more frequent for REM dream speech
Ref. 443 - p. 375

1020. EXPERIMENTS WHICH APPEAR TO DEMONSTRATE TELEPATHIC
EFFECTS IN DREAMS:
1. Have been disproven by EEG-EOG monitoring
2. Require that the agent concentrate upon the target
3. Require that the dreamer concentrate intensely prior to sleep
4. Utilize blind evaluation of target dream correspondences
Ref. 444 - p. 394

1021. THE MANIFEST DREAMS OF:
1. Alcoholics have more themes of oral incorporation than do those of
schizophrenics
2. Acute schizophrenics are more varied than those of chronic
schizophrenics
3. Normals have a greater number of positive interactions between the
dreamer and female figures
4. Suicidal patients have themes of death and destructive hostility to a
greater extent than the dreams of controls
Ref. 445 - p. 404

1022. TALENTED MALE COLLEGE DROPOUTS TEND TO:
1. Be among the more mature students
2. Have intense conflicts centering around ambivalent identifications
with their fathers
3. Have a longstanding pattern of engagement as a response to conflict
4. Form a "negative transference" to the college
Ref. 446 - p. 17

1023. RECENT RESEARCH HAS INDICATED THAT PERSONS WHO BECOME
LONG-TERM PATIENTS IN A STATE MENTAL HOSPITAL AS OPPOSED
TO THOSE WHO WERE DISCHARGED MORE QUICKLY, SHOW ON
ADMISSION:
1. A higher propensity to dependent behavior
2. Passive forms of aggression toward authority
3. Movement toward a "negative identity" (Erikson)
4. Gross psychotic symptomatology such as hallucinations, loss of
impulse control, or disordered thinking
Ref. 447 - p. 21

1024. ACCORDING TO GOFFMAN, A "TOTAL INSTITUTION" IS ONE IN WHICH
THERE IS A BREAKDOWN OF THE BARRIERS WHICH ORDINARILY
SEPARATE THE SPHERES OF:
1. Sleep
2. Play
3. Work
4. Treatment
Ref. 447 - p. 26

1025.   IN A "TOTAL INSTITUTION":
        1.   All aspects of life are conducted in the same place
        2.   There is a diversity of authority
        3.   All members are treated alike
        4.   The day's activities are loosely scheduled
                                        Ref. 447 - p. 26

1026.   HALEY APPROACHES THE PROBLEM OF DEFINING THE NATURE OF
        SCHIZOPHRENIA WITH THE CONCEPT OF:
        1.   Avoidance of the process of defining relationships
        2.   Organ language
        3.   Stripping messages of their metacommunicative meanings
        4.   Unconscious equivalent of devouring the objects
                                        Ref. 448 - p. 38

1027.   IN THE SCHIZOPHRENIC FAMILY, ACCORDING TO HALEY:
        1.   The father tends to initiate what happens
        2.   The mother accepts responsibility for the child's behavior
        3.   The children avoid household responsibility
        4.   There is a collective denial that anyone is setting the rules
                                        Ref. 488 - p. 41

1028.   THE SCHIZOPHRENIC FAMILY IS CHARACTERIZED BY HALEY AS
        POSSESSING:
        1.   A veneer of glossy hope and good intentions
        2.   Despair
        3.   A power-struggle to the death
        4.   Continual confusion   Ref. 448 - p. 43

1029.   CHARACTERISTICS OF TOTAL INSTITUTIONS THAT APPLY TO
        PATHOLOGICAL FAMILIES AND MENTAL HOSPITALS INCLUDE:
        1.   Facilitation of growth
        2.   A small group controls a larger group
        3.   There is no rationale
        4.   Inducement of guilt   Ref. 448 - p. 44

1030.   ACCORDING TO HALEY, THE THERAPIST GAINS CONTROL OF THE
        RELATIONSHIP:
        1.   By the judicious use of drugs
        2.   When the patient is hospitalized
        3.   Through anonymity
        4.   Through the posing of paradoxes
                                        Ref. 448 - p. 45

1031.   IN BION'S CONCEPT OF THE GROUP:
        1.   A group is defined as a function of an aggregate of individuals
        2.   People must come together in the same place to form a group
        3.   Two groups are present in every group
        4.   A herd instinct is postulated   Ref. 449 - p. 57

1032.   ACCORDING TO BION THE BASIC ASSUMPTION GROUPS CONSIST OF:
        1   Dependency groups
        2.   Fight-flight groups
        3.   Pairing groups
        4.   Work groups   Ref. 449 - p. 58

154

1033. IT APPEARS THAT REGULAR USERS OF MARIJUANA:
1. Eschew alcohol
2. Do not develop serious dependence on other drugs
3. Find no impairment in their driving ability
4. Have a higher rate of divorce or separation
Ref. 450 - p. 437

1034. THE MARIJUANA USER APPEARS TO BE ESPECIALLY ATTRACTED TO:
1. Sedatives
2. Antidepressants
3. Tranquilizers
4. Amphetamines
Ref. 450 - p. 441

1035. IMMEDIATELY FOLLOWING THE LOSS BY DEATH OF A SPOUSE:
1. Identification phenomena develop
2. Guilt feelings set in
3. The phase of yearning begins
4. A state of numbers sets in
Ref. 451 - p. 448

1036. IDENTIFICATION PHENOMENA WHICH DEVELOP FOLLOWING THE
DEATH OF A HUSBAND ARE CHARACTERIZED BY:
1. Behavior and thinking more like that of the husband
2. Symptoms closely resembling the symptoms of the husband's last
illness
3. Feelings that the dead husband is actually inside them
4. Location of the dead husband in their children
Ref. 451 - p. 459

1037. BOWLBY'S DESCRIPTION OF GRIEF AS A PHASIC PROCESS INCLUDES
THE PHASE OF:
1. Numbness
2. Yearning and protest
3. Disorganization
4. Elation
Ref. 451 - p. 465

1038. CORE VALUES OF THE KIBBUTZ INCLUDE:
1. Emphasis on intellectual achievement
2. Importance of the group
3. Artistic creativity
4. Conformity
Ref. 452 - p. 492

1039. IN THE PSYCHOSIS ASSOCIATED WITH MYXEDEMA:
1. Organic features are rare
2. Paranoid ideas are common
3. Memory for recent events is spared
4. The most frequent type of disturbance is a delirious-hallucinatory
reaction with clouding of consciousness
Ref. 453 - p. 3

1040. PSYCHOPATHOLOGICAL SYMPTOMS FOLLOWING HYPOTHYROIDISM:
1. Usually recede if the patient is adequately treated with thyroid hormone,
when beginning late in life
2. Often persist with intellectual reduction when hypothroidism is congenital or starts early in life
3. Often go undiagnosed for many years
4. When not complicated by psychosis are characterized by psychomotor
retardation
Ref. 453 - p. 2

1041. TYPICAL CHANGES SEEN IN THE PSYCHOSIS ASSOCIATED WITH
HYPOTHYROIDISM INCLUDE:
1. Lowering of voltage in EEG
2. Slowing of waves in EEG
3. Flattening or inversion of T waves in ECG
4. ECG that shows tachycardia   Ref. 453 - p. 11

1042. THE FREQUENCY OF TARDIVE DYSKINESIA IS INCREASED:
1. In older patients
2. In men
3. With longer duration of treatment
4. With megavitamin therapy   Ref. 454 - p. 15

1043. THE MOST FREQUENT MUSCLE GROUPS INVOLVED IN TARDIVE DYS-
KINESIA ARE THOSE OF THE:
1. Lips
2. Tongue
3. Jaw
4. Arm   Ref. 454 - p. 14

1044. DIFFERENCES IN OUTCOME IN THE COURSE OF SCHIZOPHRENIA
COULD BE EXPLAINED ON THE BASIS OF THERE BEING A TYPE
OF SCHIZOPHRENIA WHICH IS:
1. A remitting illness in which the length of remission exceeds two years
2. A relapsing illness in which episodes of remission are rarely complete
and last for less than two years
3. A rare form in which progressive deterioration seems to occur in
spite of determined treatment, both physical and psychological
4. Curable by phenothiazine treatment
                         Ref. 455 - p. 32

1045. LYMPHOCYTE ABNORMALITIES IN SCHIZOPHRENIA MAY BE RELATED
TO:
1. Phytohemagglutinin
2. Ascorbic acid deficiency
3. Taraxein
4. Phenothiazine treatment   Ref. 456 - p. 69

1046. POSTPUBERTAL BOYS WITH KLINEFELTER'S SYNDROME ARE
CHARACTERIZED BY:
1. Passivity
2. Having a positive sex chromatin pattern
3. Being tall and awkward
4. Intellectual superiority   Ref. 457 - p. 79

1047. THERE APPEARS TO BE A DISTURBANCE IN THE DOPAMINE META-
BOLISM IN THE BRAIN OF PATIENTS WITH:
1. Idiopathic parkinsonism
2. Postencephalitic parkinsonism
3. Senile dementia
4. Presenile dementia   Ref. 458 - p. 103

156

1048.   THE KLEINE-LEVIN SYNDROME:
1. Begins during adolescence
2. Occurs mainly in women
3. Eventually disappears of itself
4. Is characterized by intellectual impairment
                                        Ref. 459 - p. 106

1049.   PATIENTS WITH THE KLEINE-LEVIN SYNDROME:
1. Suffer from excessive sleepiness
2. Suffer from excessive eating
3. Have a patchy amnesia for the attack
4. Seem to respond best to amphetamine
                                        Ref. 459 - p. 109

1050.   LITHIUM CARBONATE APPEARS TO CAUSE AN INCREASE IN:
1. Bilirubin
2. WBC
3. Blood pressure
4. Body weight   Ref. 460 - p. 238

1051.   THERE IS AN INCREASE IN TOTAL BODY WATER:
1. In recovery from depression with lithium carbonate treatment
2. In recovery from mania with lithium carbonate treatment
3. In recovery from depression
4. During depression   Ref. 461 - p. 254

1052.   IN TURNER'S SYNDROME THERE OCCURS:
1. Short stature and underdeveloped secondary sex characteristics
2. Webbing of the neck
3. Deformity of the elbow
4. Lack of X chromosome material   Ref. 462 - p. 286

1053.   PATIENTS WITH TURNER'S SYNDROME:
1. Are very feminine
2. Are most often well-liked by everybody
3. Show a decrease in performance with preservation of verbal function
4. Have a high risk of mental illness
                                        Ref. 462 - p. 307

1054.   PATIENTS WITH KLINEFELTER'S SYNDROME:
1. Show a decreased verbal and a preserved performance function
2. Have a visual dysagnosia or space-form blindness
3. May manifest asocial behavior and criminality
4. Are very masculine   Ref. 462 - p. 308

1055.   SYMPTOMS WHICH ARE COMMON IN TURNER'S SYNDROME ARE:
1. Anxiety
2. Psychosis
3. Immaturity
4. Aggressiveness   Ref. 462 - p. 309

1056.   A PSYCHOTROPIC DRUG WHICH WOULD BE CONVENIENT TO BE USED
AS A PREPARATION IN DEPOT FORM FOR PROLONGED EFFECT IS:
1. Thorazine
2. Sparine
3. Mellaril
4. Fluphenazine   Ref. 463 - p. 311

1057. SIDE EFFECTS OF THE USE OF PSYCHOTROPIC DEPOT PREPARATIONS
WHICH OFTEN LEAD TO THE DRUG HAVING TO BE STOPPED INCLUDE:
1. Excessive drowsiness
2. Absence of neuroleptic effect
3. Low level of patient acceptance
4. Extra-pyramidal effects   Ref. 463 - p. 317

1058. THE "PINK SPOT":
1. Is found in Tay-Sachs disease
2. Is produced on paper chromatograms of urinary extracts
3. Has been found mainly in depressions
4. Was first demonstrated with reference to schizophrenic patients
                                     Ref. 464 - p. 374

1059. VARIOUS STUDIES HAVE IDENTIFIED THE "PINK SPOT" PRECURSOR
AS:
1. 4-methoxyphenylethylamine
2. Monoacetylcadaverine
3. P-tyramine
4. 3, 4-dimethoxyphenylethylamine   Ref. 464 - p. 375

1060. FOLIE A DEUX:
1. Generally occurs in a setting of paranoid psychosis
2. Occurs between persons of the opposite sex generally
3. Is characterized by improvement of the submissive partner upon
   separation, in the imposed form of the illness
4. Appears most often in the simultaneous type
                                     Ref. 465 - p. 413

1061. QUANTITATIVE ANALYSIS OF THE EEG DURING THE PERIOD OF
HYPNOTIC TRANCE INDUCTION REVEALS:
1. Increase of alpha activity
2. Increase amplitude
3. Decrease of slow waves
4. 14 and 6 cps waves   Ref. 466 - p. 804

1062. VARIOUS STUDIES HAVE RELATED GOOD HYPNOTIZABILITY WITH:
1. Very-high-frequency superimposed beta activity in the resting EEG
2. Increase in alpha activity
3. Increase of slow waves
4. Temporal spikes   Ref. 466 - p. 804

1063. COMPOUNDS WHICH ACCELERATE THE EEG FREQUENCIES INCLUDE:
1. Lithium
2. LSD
3. I.V. barbiturates in high doses
4. Dextroamphetamine   Ref. 466 - p. 804

1064. RECENT FINDINGS DEMONSTRATE THAT DURING THE HYPNOTIC
TRANCE THERE OCCURS ON THE EEG:
1. High voltage slow activity
2. A spike and wave pattern
3. Decreased alpha
4. Increased very-high-frequency superimposed beta activity
                                     Ref. 466 - p. 804

1065.   SUGGESTIBILITY AND HYPNOTIZABILITY ARE INCREASED BY:
1.   Thorazine
2.   LSD
3.   Tofranil
4.   Amphetamine   Ref. 466 - p. 804

1066.   AFTER CANCER PATIENTS ARE INFORMED OF THEIR DIAGNOSIS,
THE INITIAL SHOCK PHASE PROGRESSES TO THE STAGE OF:
1.   Denial
2.   Bargaining
3.   Depression
4.   Withdrawal of interest from the environment
Ref. 467 - p. 806

1067.   TREATMENT ON A CANCER WARD IS CARRIED OUT BEST WHEN:
1.   Family members are not permitted to spend long hours with the
patient
2.   Patients are discouraged from taking leaves of absence from the
hospital
3.   Discussion of their illness with patients utilizing marked denial
is minimized
4.   There is at least one person who can listen with understanding to
fears concerning death   Ref. 467 - p. 808

1068.   REGARDING THE PROBLEM OF VIOLENCE, IT HAS BEEN FOUND
THAT:
1.   The most likely murderer is a stranger
2.   Fear of criminal attack and murder exists in the minds of many
urban dwellers and is a destructive force in the deterioration of the
American city
3.   Homicide causes as many violent deaths as do automobile accidents
4.   The statistical chance of being murdered in any year is approximately
one in 20,000   Ref. 468 - p. 811

1069.   MURDERS IN THE UNITED STATES:
1.   Have a rate over ten times that of Great Britain
2.   Have robbery as their most frequent motive when committed by
strangers
3.   Are committed with a gun in the majority of cases
4.   Have been decreasing in rate since the mid-1960s
Ref. 468 - p. 812

1070.   IN THE VIDEOTAPE METHOD OF PSYCHOTHERAPY SUPERVISION:
1.   The therapist should take notes during the session
2.   The expense of the system is minimal
3.   The supervisor should stop the tape every few moments and comment
4.   The therapist can observe his own nonverbal behavior
Ref. 469 - p. 821

1071.   ASPECTS OF THINKING WHICH HAVE BEEN USED AS INDICES OF A
SCHIZOPHRENIC THOUGHT DISORDER INCLUDE:
1.   Overinclusiveness
2.   Underinclusiveness
3.   Bizarre idiosyncratic quality
4.   Originality   Ref. 470 - p. 825

1072   ON THE PROGNOSTIC INDEX FOR PREDICTION OF OUTCOME IN
        PSYCHOTHERAPY, FAVORABLE SIGNS ARE:
        1. Anxiety and depression
        2. Early environmental trauma
        3. Recognizable precipitating event
        4. Habitual use of self-defeating patterns
                                        Ref. 471 - p. 831

1073.   THE OUTCOME OF PSYCHOTHERAPY IS SIGNIFICANTLY PREDICTED
        BY THE PROGNOSTIC INDEX BY THE SCORES ON THE FACTORS OF:
        1. General Emotional Health
        2. Intellectual Achievement
        3. Acute Depression
        4. Aptitude for Psychotherapy   Ref. 471 - p. 834

1074.   APTITUDE FOR PSYCHOTHERAPY IS HIGHER IN PATIENTS WITH
        HIGH LEVELS OF:
        1. Motivation
        2. Insight
        3. Anxiety tolerance
        4. Absence of secondary gain   Ref. 471 - p. 834

1075.   DRUG ADDICTS ARE TREATED BY A SELF-HELP DAY CARE CENTER
        WITHOUT METHADONE IN:
        1. Daytop
        2. Exodus House
        3. The New York State Narcotic Program
        4. Reality House   Ref. 472 - p. 847

1076.   A CLOSED RESIDENTIAL SETTING FOR THE TREATMENT OF HEROIN
        ADDICTION WITHOUT METHADONE IS:
        1. Synanon
        2. Phoenix House
        3. Odyssey House
        4. Esalen   Ref. 472 - p. 847

1077.   THE USE OF HARSH, DEVASTATING CONFRONTATIONS AND THE
        STRIPPING OF THE PATIENT RAPIDLY TO THE LEVEL OF HELP-
        LESSNESS IS CHARACTERISTIC OF THE TREATMENT PROGRAM OF:
        1. Synanon
        2. Reality House
        3. Daytop
        4. The Narcotic Addict Rehabilitation Act Program
                                        Ref. 472 - p. 851

1078.   THE NARCOTIC ADDICT REHABILITATION ACT PASSED BY CONGRESS
        IN 1966:
        1. Provides for the establishment of methadone maintenance clinics in
            the cities in which addiction is common
        2. Authorizes commitment for treatment of addicts charged with
            certain crimes who elect treatment rather than prosecution
        3. Has led to a reduction in the magnitude of the addiction problem
            and attendant criminal activity
        4. Provides for civil commitment for six months hospitalization
            followed by compulsory supervised after care for 36 months
                                        Ref. 473 - p. 853

1079. THE TYPICAL SUCCESSFUL PATIENT IN THE NARCOTIC ADDICT
    REHABILITATION ACT PROGRAM, IN CONTRAST TO THE UNSUCCESS-
    FUL PATIENT, IS:
    1. White
    2. A high school graduate
    3. One who lived with both parents until the age of six
    4. Under greater external pressure to comply with the treatment
    Ref. 473 - p. 855

1080. MAJOR ELEMENTS OF THE NARCOTICS TREATMENT ADMINISTRATION
    PROGRAM OF WASHINGTON D.C. INCLUDE:
    1. Methadone maintenance
    2. Ex-addict counselors
    3. Self-referrals and court-referrals
    4. Primary emphasis on inpatient treatment
    Ref. 474 - p. 857

SELECT THE MOST APPROPRIATE COMPLETION IN THE FOLLOWING
MULTIPLE CHOICE QUESTIONS:

1081. THE BADEN FORMULA FOR THE ESTIMATIONS OF THE NUMBER OF
    HEROIN ADDICTS IS BASED ON:
    A. The number of arrest for possession
    B. Overdose deaths
    C. Police department statistics for robberies and muggings
    D. Information obtained from police informants
    E. The total population at risk   Ref. 474 - p. 857

1082. A GOOD PROGNOSTICATOR FOR SUCCESSFUL RENUNCIATION OF
    HEROIN-ADDICTION IS:
    A. Occurrence of sudden traumatic incidents coinciding with onset of
       drug abuse
    B. Precocious sexual experiences
    C. "Burning out"
    D. Close relationship with the mother
    E. Absence of prostitution history   Ref. 475 - p. 862

1083. IN THE TREATMENT OF THE DRUG ADDICT IT IS CRUCIAL THAT
    THERE BE:
    A. Screening to find those addicts who are most apt to renounce drugs
    B. Continued long-term supervision
    C. Counseling to encourage higher aspirational levels
    D. Realistic educational and employment opportunities
    E. All of the above   Ref. 475 - p. 864

1084. IN AN ADDICTION TREATMENT PROGRAM, THOSE PATIENTS WHO
    ARE SUCCESSFUL IN RENOUNCING DRUG USE TEND TO:
    A. Be among the more severely disturbed
    B. Have shown antisocial behavior prominently prior to addiction
    C. Have grown up in broken homes
    D. Have had fathers who provided suitable models for work roles
    E. All of the above   Ref. 475 - p. 861

1085. THE TREATMENT OF THE HEROIN ADDICT IN THE WALK-IN
PSYCHIATRIC CLINIC OF A GENERAL HOSPITAL IS SIGNIFICANTLY
IMPROVED BY THE USE OF:
A. Psychotropic medication
B. Individual and group therapy
C. Methadone detoxification
D. All of the above
E. None of the above   Ref. 476 - p. 865

1086. ELEVATED RATIO OF CORTICOID TO ANDROGENIC STEROIDS IN
WOMEN IS CORRELATED WITH POOR PROGNOSIS IN:
A. Regional ileitis
B. Ulcerative colitis
C. Lupus erythematosus
D. Cancer of the breast
E. Bronchial asthma   Ref. 477 - p. 16

1087. A HIGHLY SIGNIFICANT COVARIANCE HAS BEEN FOUND BETWEEN
HYDROCORTISONE PRODUCTION RATE AND:
A. Depression
B. Anxiety
C. Thinking disorder
D. Motivation for treatment
E. Extend of defensive failing   Ref. 477 - p. 1

1088. ELEVATION IN BLOOD PRESSURE HAS BEEN FOUND TO OCCUR IN MEN:
A. Who experience job loss
B. Upon entering the armed forces
C. Who are about to graduate from college
D. Who have recently married
E. During the wife's pregnancy   Ref. 478 - p. 36

1089. THE MOST CONSISTENT AND RELIABLE METHOD OF MEASURING A
SUBJECT'S ESTIMATION OF A TIME INTERVAL IS:
A. Verbal estimation
B. Production
C. Reproduction
D. Comparison
E. None of the above   Ref. 479 - p. 41

1090. VARIATIONS IN TIME PERCEPTION OCCUR UNDER THE INFLUENCE OF:
A. Thyroid hormone
B. Cortisol levels
C. Diurnal changes
D. The menstrual cycle
E. All of the above   Ref. 479 - p. 40

1091. CORTISOL ADMINISTRATION CAUSES A SIGNIFICANT DECREASE IN:
A. Two-flash fusion threshold
B. Score on Mood Adjective Check List
C. Alpha-rhythm frequency
D. Amplitude of average evoked potential
E. Produced estimates of 60-second intervals
          Ref. 479 - p. 48

1092. DRIVE THEORIES OF SCHIZOPHRENIA SHARE IN COMMON THE
ASSUMPTION THAT A BASIC DEFECT IN SCHIZOPHRENIA CONSISTS IN:
A. Lack of motivation for interpersonal interaction
B. Weakness of libidinal cathexes
C. Low threshold for disorganization under increasing stimulus input
D. Difficulty in neutralization of aggressive drives
E. Heightened instinctual drives   Ref. 480 - p. 137

1093. FOR PAVLOV, THE TWO PROCESSES, THE INTERACTION OF WHICH
ACCOUNTS FOR ALL BEHAVIOR, ARE:
A. Primary and secondary processes
B. Excitation and inhibition
C. Activation and neutralization
D. Cathexes and countercathexes
E. Drive and defense   Ref. 480 - p. 124

1094. IN PAVLOV'S THEORY, THE SYMPTOMS OF SCHIZOPHRENIA ARE
ATTRIBUTED TO:
A. Excitatory modulation
B. Input dysfunction
C. Response strength ceiling
D. Transmarginal inhibition
E. Reciprocal augmentation   Ref. 480 - p. 124

MATCH EACH DRIVE THEORY OF SCHIZOPHRENIA WITH THE
RELATED MECHANISM:

A. Reciprocal Augmentation of anxiety and Stimulus Generalization
B. Response Strength Ceiling
C. Input Dysfunction
D. Transmarginal Inhibition
E. Disorder of Excitatory Modulation

1095. ___ Defect in breadth of attention   Ref. 480 -
1096. ___ Primary symptoms produced by a state of heightened drive; self-
perpetuating spiral
1097. ___ Inhibition of internal inhibition accounting for regression, inability
to delay, inability to maintain a set, and breakdown in discrimination
1098. ___ Tendency of schizophrenic to over- or under-respond
1099. ___ Associative disturbance produced by appropriate and inappropriate
tendencies having nearly equal probabilities of occurrence
          Ref. 480 - pp. 114,117,121,
                              127,130

1100. THE LAW OF EXCITATORY MODULATION:
A. States that the gradient of inhibition is steeper than the gradient of excitation
B. Explains why the organism can respond to rapid rates of stimulation without being overwhelmed
C. Assumes that the expansion of the gradients of inhibition and excitation produce an   expansion of awareness without a corresponding increase in excitability
D. All of the above
E. None of the above   Ref. 480 - p. 128

1101. THE THEORY OF UNASSIMILATED PERCEPTS:
A. Attempts to explain schizophrenic symptoms
B. Is primarily a cognitive theory with secondary implications for arousal
C. Assumes that anxiety is produced when experience cannot be interpreted into conceptual schemata
D. All of the above
E. None of the above   Ref. 480 - p. 134

1102. PATIENTS WITH AMYOTROPHIC LATERAL SCLEROSIS:
A. Usually have had a characteristic life style and anxiety and depression
B. Have reversal of their insulin resistance and decreased glucose utilization by treatment with amitriptyline
C. Rarely demonstrate calm and detachment toward their debilitating illness
D. All of the above
E. None of the above   Ref. 481 - p. 141

1103. AFTER TOTAL SLEEP DEPRIVATION, SUBJECTS SHOW:
A. Recovery of stage 4 sleep before REM sleep
B. Increase above base line levels of REM sleep on first recovery night
C. Delay in increase of stage 4 sleep until the second and third recovery nights
D. Increase in stage 2 and 3 before stage 4
E. No increase in stage 4 sleep   Ref. 482 - p. 189

1104. FOLLOWING PROLONGED   (205 HOURS) SLEEP DEPRIVATION SUBJECTS DEMONSTRATE:
A. The recovery pattern sequence unchanged
B. The recovery pattern sequence reversed
C. REM sleep increase before stage 4 increase
D. Stage 4 increase before REM sleep increase
E. Increase in both REM sleep and stage 4 sleep on the first recovery night   Ref. 482 - p. 198

1105. IN TOTAL STARVATION FOR THE TREATMENT OF SEVERE OBESITY:
A. There is a weight loss of approximately one pound daily
B. Physical sensations of hunger persist for the duration of fasting
C. A metabolic alkalosis ensues caused by the breakdown of fats
D. Intake of vitamins, fluids and electrolyte replacement is usually unnecessary
E. Normal physical activity is discouraged
Ref. 483 - p. 209

1106.   STUDIES OF SUPEROBESE PATIENTS STARVED FOR OBESITY
        TREATMENT REVEAL:
        A.   Fewer psychological problems are present
        B.   Weight lost in the hospital tends to be maintained
        C.   Modification of appetite and intake on a long term basis
        D.   All of the above
        E.   None of the above   Ref. 483 - p. 213

1107.   THE CAPACITY OF ONE-YEAR OLD INFANTS TO MAINTAIN THEIR
        INTEREST IN THE FACE OF FRUSTRATION IN AN EXPERIMENTAL
        SITUATION:
        A.   Is higher in males than in females
        B.   Is equal in males and females
        C.   Is higher in females than in males
        D.   Is not measurable
        E.   Has no significance   Ref. 484 - p. 255

1108.   IN THE ADRENOGENITAL SYNDROME, SEX CHANGE:
        A.   Should not be considered after the age of 2
        B.   May revert a pseudohermaphrodite into reproductive female
        C.   Should be postponed to later childhood
        D.   Cannot be performed
        E.   None of the above   Ref. 485 - p. 460

1109.   THE SMOKING OF CIGARETTES:
        A.   Occurs in 50% of the adult males in the United States
        B.   Leads to a state of physiological dependence having withdrawal
             effects that can be aborted by nicotine
        C.   Correlates positively with the use of opiates, alcohol, and marijuana
        D.   All of the above
        E.   None of the above   Ref. 486 - p. 482,484

1110.   DURING PERIODS OF SMOKING DEPRIVATION, THE FOLLOWING
        OCCUR, EXCEPT:
        A.   Dysphoria
        B.   Perceptual disturbance
        C.   Drowsiness
        D.   Restlessness
        E.   Increase in slow wave EEG activity
                                          Ref. 486 - p. 484

1111.   HEAVY SMOKERS ARE CHARACTERIZED BY THE FOLLOWING,
        EXCEPT:
        A.   Compliance
        B.   Impulsiveness
        C.   Danger-seeking
        D.   Emotional lability
        E.   Oral preoccupation   Ref. 486 - p. 469

1112.   WOMEN WHO HAVE A POOR POSTPARTUM ADJUSTMENT, SHOW
        THE FOLLOWING ON THEIR ANTEPARTUM RORSCHACH AND TAT:
        A.   Higher ratio of female to male percents
        B.   Greater preoccupation with their pregnancy
        C.   Higher number of themes relating to acceptance of maternal role
        D.   Higher number of themes relating to acceptance of feminine role
        E.   All of the above   Ref. 487 - p. 492

1113.   THE VISUAL AVERAGE EVOKED POTENTIAL (AEP):
    A.   Is enhanced in amplitude when the subject attends to pattern
         reversals of the background
    B.   Is decreased in amplitude when the subject attends to a certain
         stimulus
    C.   Is a measure of the subject's ability to attend selectively to
         significant stimuli
    D.   All of the above
    E.   None of the above   Ref. 488 - p. 496

1114.   SUBJECTS WITH CORONARY HEART DISEASE ARE FOUND TO:
    A.   Be highly passive
    B.   Avoid competition
    C.   Strive against time deadlines
    D.   Be decreasing in incidence
    E.   Have few marital problems   Ref. 489 - p. 524

1115.   IN A STUDY OF IDENTICAL MALE TWINS DISCORDANT FOR CORONARY
        HEART DISEASE, INTRAPAIR CHD DIFFERENCES CORRELATE WITH
        DIFFERENCES IN:
    A.   Cigarette smoking history
    B.   Blood pressure
    C.   Serum cholesterol
    D.   FBS
    E.   Life dissatisfactions   Ref. 489 - p. 537

1116.   SUBJECTS, IN THE ABOVE STUDY, WITH RELATIVELY SEVERE CHD:
    A.   Described poor childhood interpersonal relations
    B.   Described poor adult interpersonal relations
    C.   Felt they had too low a level of income
    D.   Regretted their working conditions
    E.   Had relatively higher educational levels
                                      Ref. 489 - p. 535

1117.   A GOOD PROGNOSIS FOR PSYCHOANALYTIC PSYCHOTHERAPY IN
        PATIENTS FUNCTIONING ON AN OVERTLY BORDERLINE LEVEL IS
        FOUND IN THOSE WHOSE PERSONALITY IS:
    A.   Hysterical
    B.   Schizoid
    C.   Narcissistic
    D.   All of the above
    E.   None of the above   Ref. 490 - p. 598

1118.   A BAD PROGNOSIS FOR PSYCHOANALYTIC PSYCHOTHERAPY IN
        PATIENTS FUNCTIONING ON A BORDERLINE LEVEL IS FOUND IN:
    A.   Hypomanic personalities
    B.   Impulse-ridden character disorders
    C.   Obsessive-compulsive personalities
    D.   All of the above
    E.   None of the above   Ref. 490 - p. 603

1119. THE WORST PROGNOSIS FOR ANY KIND OF PSYCHOLOGICAL
       TREATMENT IS FOUND IN:
       A. Depressive personalities
       B. Paranoid personalities
       C. Antisocial personalities
       D. Patients suffering from sexual deviations
       E. Patients suffering from alcohol and drug addiction
                                              Ref. 490 - p. 622

1120. THE SKILL OF THE THERAPIST IS THE MOST CRUCIAL FACTOR IN
       THE OUTCOME OF TREATMENT:
       A. Of patients with high ego strength
       B. Of patients with low ego strength
       C. Which forces the therapist into a position of rather strict neutrality
       D. Which is expressive rather than supportive
       E. None of the above   Ref. 490 - p. 630

1121. A FUNDAMENTAL PROGNOSTIC FACTOR IN THE TREATMENT OF
       PATIENTS WITH BORDERLINE PERSONALITY ORGANIZATION IS:
       A. Capacity for depression and guilt
       B. Anxiety tolerance
       C. Impulse control
       D. Sublimatory potential
       E. All of the above   Ref. 490 - p. 625, 613

1122. IN SPITE OF THEIR SURPRISINGLY GOOD SURFACE FUNCTION IN
       SOCIAL GROUPS, POOR OBJECT RELATIONS ARE CHARACTERISTIC
       OF:
       A. Hysterical personalities
       B. Antisocial personalities
       C. Narcissistic personalities
       E. Borderline patients   Ref. 490 - p. 629

1123. WHEN A PSYCHOTHERAPIST BECOMES AWARE THAT A PATIENT IS
       LYING TO HIM, THE PROPER RESPONSE IS:
       A. No response until patient spontaneously acknowledges the lying
       B. Cautious suggestion that the truth is being avoided
       C. Interpretation of the patient's unconscious hostility
       D. Confrontation
       E. Termination   Ref. 490 - p. 625

1124. PERSONALITY CHARACTERISTICS OF THE THERAPIST WHICH ARE
       UNDESIRABLE FOR THE TREATMENT OF BORDERLINE CASES INCLUDE
       THE FOLLOWING, EXCEPT:
       A. Clear sense of moral values
       B. Unconcern regarding acting out
       C. Retention of his own narcissism
       D. Overconcern regarding acting out
       E. Lowered capacity for sustaining object-relationships under
           frustrating conditions   Ref. 490 - p. 632

1125. DURING THE PROCESS OF MOURNING, THE FOLLOWING OCCUR,
       EXCEPT:
       A. Emotional pain
       B. Denial
       C. Loss of interest in the outside world
       D. Loss of the capacity to adopt any new object of love
       E. Reality testing   Ref. 491 - p. 698

1126. AFTER THE LOSS OF A PARENT PRIOR TO ADOLESCENCE THERE
OCCURS THE FOLLOWING, EXCEPT:
A. Continuation of immersion in the activities of everyday life
B. Withdrawal into preoccupation with thoughts of the lost parent
C. Denying the finality of the loss
D. Sad feelings and weeping in curtailed forms
E. Occasional good moods   Ref. 491 - p. 701, 703

1127. THE MOST INTENSE AFFECT EXPERIENCED BY BEREAVED CHILDREN
IS:
A. Grief
B. Sadness
C. Anxiety
D. Rage
E. Guilt   Ref. 491 - p. 704

1128. THE CONCEPT OF THE EGO IS BEST DEFINED AS:
A. An actual part of the brain
B. An anthropomorphic executor
C. The functional part of the self
D. A group of functions
E. The self   Ref. 492 - p. 772

1129. ACCORDING TO MAHLER, THE DEVELOPMENTAL-MATURATIONAL
PHASE IN WHICH OBJECT CONSTANCY IS ACHIEVED IS THE:
A. Depressed phase
B. Paranoid phase
C. Autistic phase
D. Symbiotic phase
E. Separation-individuation phase   Ref. 493 - p. 789

1130. ACCORDING TO MAHLER'S OBSERVATION'S, THERE OCCURS DURING
THE PRACTICING PERIOD PAR EXCELLENCE (9th - 18th MONTH):
A. A gradual unfolding of the Oedipus complex
B. The development of the superego
C. A basic mood of elation
D. The basis for later moods of depression
E. The roots of anxiety   Ref. 493 - p. 789

1131. THE TERM "HESPERIAN DEPRESSION" REFERS TO:
A. Mood changes triggered by the dusk
B. Depression which follows occupational success
C. Postpartum affective disturbance
D. Early morning depression
E. Schizophrenic depression   Ref. 494 - p. 805

1132. THE ABILITY TO DISTINGUISH THE LOVE OBJECT FROM ALL
OTHER OBJECTS MAY BE THE BASIS OF:
A. The smiling response
B. Attention
C. Stranger anxiety
D. Preperception
E. Perception   Ref. 495 - p. 441

1133. THE ABOVE PHENOMENON USUALLY BEGINS AT AGE:
A. One months
B. Three months
C. Four months
D. Eight months
E. One year   Ref. 495 - p. 441

1134. NARCISSISTIC PERSONALITIES:
A. Do not benefit from psychoanalysis
B. Do not establish a transference relationship
C. Do not associate freely
D. All of the above
E. None of the above   Ref. 496 - p. 452

1135. MOST INVESTIGATORS AGREE THAT THE SPIDER IN SPIDER PHOBIAS IS A REPRESENTATION OF:
A. The sibling rival
B. The hated father
C. The dangerous mother
D. Castration anxiety
E. Penis envy   Ref. 497 - p. 493

1136. THE SOURCE OF A DREAM IS:
A. A recent and significant event represented in the dream directly
B. Several recent and significant experiences combined into a single unity by the dream
C. Recent and significant experiences represented in the dream by mention of a contemporary but indifferent experience
D. An internal significant experience (a memory of train of thought) invariably represented by a mention of a recent but indifferent impression
E. All of the above   Ref. 498 - p. 501

1137. THE TYPE OF THOUGHT IMPULSE WHICH PERSISTS IN SLEEP IS:
A. What has not been carried to a conclusion during the day
B. What has not been solved
C. What has been suppressed during the day
D. Indifferent impressions which for that reason have not been dealt with
E. All of the above   Ref. 498 - p. 502

1138. IT IS WELL TO BEGIN THE EXPLORATION OF A DREAM BY:
A. Presenting the therapist's associations
B. Interpreting the transference implications
C. Dealing with the symbolic content
D. Asking for the day residues
E. Silence   Ref. 498 - p. 504

1139. ACCORDING TO BAK, THE BASIS OF ALL PERVERSIONS IS:
A. Oral frustration
B. The symbiotic mother
C. The masochistic position
D. The fantasy of the hidden female phallus
E. Narcissistic mortification   Ref. 499 - p. 311

1140.   A CRITERION FOR THE TERMINATION OF AN ANALYSIS IS THE:
        A. Capacity for a full trust of the analyst
        B. Increased capacity for candor on the part of the patient
        C. Increased capacity for candor on the part of the analyst
        D. Patient's ability to remain unruffled by his analyst
        E. All of the above   Ref. 500 - p. 339

        SELECT THE SLEEP STAGE THAT IS ASSOCIATED WITH THE LISTED
        SLEEP CHARACTERISTICS:

        A. Stage I - REM
        B. Stage II
        C. Stage III - IV
        D. All of the above
        E. None of the above

1141. ___ Makes up about 50% of total sleep time
1142. ___ No mental activity has been shown to occur during this stage
1143. ___ Dream reports have been recovered from 80-90% of arousals from
        this stage
1144. ___ EEG is characterized by large slow waves
1145. ___ Occurs during the first few hours of the night
1146. ___ Considerable physiological activation and fluctuation, with heart and
        respiratory rate increasing and becoming highly variable
1147. ___ Enuresis, somnambulism and night terror (pavor nocturnus) take place
        during arousal   Ref. 501 - pp. 749,750

        SELECT THE MOST APPROPRIATE COMPLETION TO THE
        FOLLOWING MULTIPLE CHOICE QUESTIONS:

1148.   FOLLOWING AROUSAL FROM SOMNAMBULISM OR PAVOR
        NOCTURNUS, THERE IS:
        A. A relatively clear sensorium
        B. Heightened reactivity to external stimuli
        C. Poor response to efforts to provoke behavioral wakefulness
        D. Clear memory for intercurrent events
        E. Good recall of the episode   Ref. 501 - p. 750

1149.   ANXIETY IS MOST SEVERE IN:
        A. The stage IV arousal reaction nightmare
        B. The REM anxiety dream when characterized as a nightmare
        C. The stage II arousal reaction
        D. The last dream of the night
        E. The hypnagogic state   Ref. 501 - p. 773

1150.   SUBJECTS WITH STAGE IV NIGHTMARES:
        A. Have a normal respiratory and heart rate in the minute just preceding
            the violent onset of the nightmare
        B. Have a very quiet and peaceful REM sleep
        C. Are frequently propelled out of bed
        D. All of the above
        E. None of the above   Ref. 501 - p. 754

1151.   MOST FRIGHTENING AROUSALS EXPERIENCED AS NIGHTMARES:
         A. Occur during Stage IV
         B. Are associated with marked vocalization or cries
         C. Are REM anxiety dreams of varying degrees of intensity
         D. Are associated with delta activity in the EEG
         E. Are preceded by an increase in heart and respiratory rate
                                               Ref. 501 - p. 757

1152.   IN NAZI CONCENTRATION CAMP SURVIVORS, NIGHTMARES:
         A. Are unrelated to the camp experience
         B. May be brought on by physiological discomfort or anxiety
         C. Are rarely experienced after the first decade
         D. All of the above
         E. None of the above   Ref. 501 - p. 770

1153.   FENICHEL SUGGESTED THAT REACTIVE TYPES OF CHARACTER
         DISORDERS BE SUBDIVIDED INTO THE FOLLOWING, EXCEPT:
         A. Phobic and hysterical characters
         B. Compulsive characters
         C. Cyclic characters
         D. Schizoid characters
         E. Sublimatory characters   Ref. 501 - p. 802

1154.   THE DIFFERENTIAL DIAGNOSIS BETWEEN PATIENTS IN THE BORDER-
         LINE FIELD AND THE PSYCHOSIS CENTERS AROUND:
         A. The mechanism of splitting
         B. Persistence of repression
         C. Persistence of reality testing
         D. Lack of anxiety tolerance
         E. Lack of impulse control   Ref. 502 - p. 810

1155.   AT THE LOWER LEVEL OF ORGANIZATION OF CHARACTER
         PATHOLOGY ONE WOULD TEND TO FIND:
         A. Hysterical characters
         B. Depressive-masochistic characters
         C. Passive-aggressive personalities
         D. Sadomasochistic personalities
         E. Antisocial personalities   Ref. 502 - p. 809

1156.   AT THE HIGHER LEVEL OF ORGANIZATION OF CHARACTER
         PATHOLOGY ONE WOULD TEND TO FIND:
         A. Hysterical characters
         B. Obsessive-compulsive characters
         C. Depressive-masochistic characters
         D. All of the above
         E. None of the above   Ref. 502 - p. 806

1157.   AT THE INTERMEDIATE LEVEL OF ORGANIZATION OF CHARACTER
         PATHOLOGY ONE WOULD TEND TO FIND:
         A. Depressive-masochistic characters
         B. Passive-aggressive personalities
         C. Antisocial personalities
         D. Inadequate personalities
         E. "As-if" characters   Ref. 502 - p. 807

1158. THE MECHANISM OF "SPLITTING" IS AN ESSENTIAL DEFENSIVE
       OPERATION OF:
       A. Hysterics
       B. Obsessionals
       C. The borderline patient
       D. Passive-aggressive personalities
       E. Neurosis   Ref. 502 - p. 811

1159. ACCORDING TO MAHLER, IN SOME TODDLERS A BASIC DEPRESSIVE
       MOOD MAY DEVELOP ARISING FROM EXPERIENCES ASSOCIATED
       WITH:
       A. Toilet training
       B. Sibling birth
       C. Discovery of sex differences
       D. All of the above
       E. None of the above   Ref. 503 - p. 846

1160. THE ABOVE NEGATIVE MOOD MANIFESTS ITSELF IN THE FOLLOWING,
       EXCEPT:
       A. Hostile dependency on the mother
       B. Frequent temper tantrums
       C. Refusal to accept temporary maternal substitution
       D. Marasmus
       E. Increasing angriness   Ref. 503 - p. 847

1161. IN A DREAM, THE REPRESENTATION OF A STATE OF MIND INSTEAD
       OF AN OBJECT IS KNOWN AS THE:
       A. Hypnoid state
       B. Hypnopompic state
       C. Functional phenomenon
       D. Material phenomenon
       E. Condensation   Ref. 504 - p. 525

1162. IN STERN'S THERAPEUTIC PLAYBACK TECHNIQUE:
       A. The new recording automatically erases that of the previous session
       B. The tape remains the property of the therapist
       C. The process is applied mainly in the treatment of borderline patients
       D. The method is introduced when treatment is begun
       E. All of the above   Ref. 505 - p. 563

1163. THE CLITORAL ORGASM:
       A. Has a sharp rise and drop like that of a man
       B. Is experienced with minimal intensity
       C. Is localized deep inside the pelvis
       D. All of the above
       E. None of the above   Ref. 506 - p. 273

1164. THE VAGINAL ORGASM:
       A. Radiates to the entire body
       B. Is characterized by a slow rise and fall
       C. Is felt deep inside the pelvis
       D. All of the above
       E. None of the above   Ref. 506 - p. 273

1165. THE INFANT WHO HAS HAD ADEQUATE HANDLING BY THE ADULTS
AROUND HIM:
   A. Is more likely to focus on the oral zone
   B. Begins to play with his genitals within the first 18 months
   C. Requires more limit-setting
   D. All of the above
   E. None of the above   Ref. 506 - p. 278

1166. FREUD DEFINED PSYCHOANALYSIS AS:
   A. A procedure for the investigation of mental processes
   B. A method for the treatment of neurotic disorders
   C. A collection of psychological information
   D. All of the above
   E. None of the above   Ref. 507 - p. 4

1167. ACCORDING TO KUHN. SCIENTIFIC ACHIEVEMENTS THAT ARE
SIMULTANEOUSLY UNPRECEDENTED AND OPEN-ENDED ARE KNOWN
AS:
   A. Innovations
   B. Paradigms
   C. Matrices
   D. Disciplines
   E. Professions   Ref. 507 - p. 4

1168. THE FOCAL DANGER IN PSYCHOSIS IS FEAR OF:
   A. Separation
   B. Castration
   C. Disintegration of the self
   D. Strangers
   E. Retribution   Ref. 508 - p. 26

1169. IN NEUROSIS, THE MAIN PROBLEM IS:
   A. Handling the instinctual demands
   B. Preservation of the self
   C. Control of acting-out
   D. The loss of identity
   E. Warding of depression   Ref. 508 - p. 27

1170. IN CONTRAST TO THE PSYCHOTIC, THE PSYCHOTIC CHARACTER:
   A. Retains a capacity to test reality
   B. Shows a push toward differentiation and maturation
   C. Has psychotic symptoms which are transitory and can be reversed
   D. All of the above
   E. None of the above   Ref. 508 - p. 48

1171. NARCISSISTIC PERSONALITIES:
   A. Do not envy others
   B. Are more impulsive than infantile personalities
   C. Have a striking capacity for empathy for the feelings of others
   D. Have an inflated concept of themselves and an inadequate need for
      tribute from others
   E. None of the above   Ref. 509 - p. 52

1172. WHAT DISTINGUISHES MANY PATIENTS WITH NARCISSISTIC PERSON-
ALITIES FROM THE USUAL BORDERLINE PATIENTS IS THEIR:
A. Defensive organization
B. Relatively good social functioning
C. Intelligence
D. Poor impulse control
E. Lack of the capacity for active and consistent work in certain areas
Ref. 509 - p. 53

1173. THE CONCEPTS OF PSYCHIC ENERGY AND CATHEXIS ARE FOUND
AT THE LEVEL OF:
A. Observational data
B. Clinical interpretation
C. Clinical generalization
D. Clinical theory
E. Metapsychology   Ref. 510 - p. 129

1174. THE CONCEPTS OF REPRESSION, DEFENSE, AND REGRESSIONS ARE:
A. Observational data
B. Clinical interpretations
C. Clinical theory
D. Metapsychological concepts
E. None of the above   Ref. 510 - p. 129

1175. REGARDING THE SEAT PREFERENCE OF PATIENTS IN GROUP
THERAPY, IT HAS BEEN SUGGESTED THAT THE FOLLOWING ARE
TRUE, EXCEPT:
A. Sitting near the door expresses alienation from the group and the
desire to leave it
B. Sofas are preferred by neurotic patients
C. Members who sit near the therapist are dependent or ingratiating
D. Members who sit at a distance from the therapist do so because
of hostility
E. The more central seats are chosen by members inclined to dominate
the discussion   Ref. 511 - p. 78

1176. HIGH VARIABILITY IN SEAT CHOICE IN GROUP PSYCHOTHERAPY
CORRELATES POSITIVELY WITH HIGH SCORES IN:
A. Motivation
B. Progress
C. Absenteeism
D. Domination
E. Dependence   Ref. 511 - p. 85

1177. IN RECENT LARGE SCALE SURVEYS OF MARIJUANA USE AMONG
HIGH SCHOOL STUDENTS, THE LOWEST PERCENTAGE USING THE
DRUG WAS FOUND IN THE STUDENTS IN:
A. Utah
B. Maryland
C. Wisconsin
D. Suburban New York City
E. California   Ref. 512 - p. 28

174

1178. IN THE MERIT SURVEY OF MARIJUANA USE IN 22,000 ABLE HIGH
SCHOOL JUNIORS AND SENIORS, IT WAS FOUND THAT:
A. The incidence figures are lower than for the general high school
population
B. Marijuana use is more common in suburban and urban communities
C. Marijuana use is highest in the Northeast states
D. All of the above
E. None of the above   Ref. 512 - p. 29

1179. MONKEYS WHO HAVE BEEN REARED FROM BIRTH IN ISOLATION
MANIFEST THE FOLLOWING, EXCEPT:
A. Hypersexuality
B. Brutal or indifferent maternal behavior
C. Minimal grooming responses
D. Self-clasping, rocking and huddling in a corner
E. Inappropriate aggression   Ref. 513 - p. 927

1180. REVERSAL OF THE EFFECTS OF ISOLATION ON MONKEYS HAS BEEN
ACCOMPLISHED THROUGH THE USE OF:
A. Antidepressant drugs
B. Emergence adaptation
C. Tranquilizers
D. Monkey therapist
E. Human therapist   Ref. 513 - p. 927

1181. THE DIFFERENCE BETWEEN A HEALTH MAINTENANCE ORGANIZA-
TION AND A COMMUNITY MENTAL HEALTH CENTER IS:
A. The HMO limits its concern to non-psychiatric conditions
B. The CMHC rarely collaborates with other community resources
C. The HMO seeks out certain high risk populations that might not seek
help even when facilities are available
D. The HMO limits its concern to the individuals of an enrolled population
E. The HMO assumes responsibility for the health of the entire
population of a geographically defined area.
Ref. 514 - p. 923

1182. PROTOTYPES OF THE HMO INCLUDE THE FOLLOWING, EXCEPT:
A. Prepaid group practice plans
B. Group Health Cooperative of Puget Sound
C. The six Kaiser plans
D. Health Insurance Plan of Greater New York (HIP)
E. Group Health Insurance (GHI)   Ref. 514 - p. 920

1183. IN A STUDY OF PERSONS SEEN IN A CHILD GUIDANCE CLINIC 30
YEARS EARLIER, THE FACTOR MOST CLEARLY CONNECTED WITH
THE DEVELOPMENT OF A SOCIOPATHIC PERSONALITY IN ADULT-
HOOD WAS:
A. Living in a slum
B. Low social class
C. Broken home
D. Sociopathy or alcoholism in the father
E. Poverty   Ref. 515 - p. 1045

1184.	THE COMMON-LAW CRITERION FOR COMPETENCY FOR TRIAL IS:
    A.	Does the defendant know the nature of the proceedings against him
    B.	Does he know his position with reference to such proceedings
    C.	Can he rationally assist counsel in his defense
    D.	All of the above
    E.	None of the above Ref. 516 - p. 1092

1185.	LITHIUM TREATMENT IN MANIA:
    A.	Produces a "chemical straight-jacketing" effect
    B.	Requires five to ten days before effects are achieved
    C.	No longer requires monitoring of serum levels
    D.	Results in a tremor which responds to antiparkinsonism agents
    E.	Restricts the emotional range Ref. 517 - pp. 377-382

1186.	A CONTRAINDICATION FOR LITHIUM TREATMENT IS THE PRESENCE OF:
    A.	Daily regimen of diuretics or continuous low-salt intake
    B.	Depression
    C.	Diabetes
    D.	Hypertension
    E.	All of the above Ref. 517 - p. 382

1187.	THE ACTION OF CHLORPROMAZINE ON THE BRAIN IS TO:
    A.	Stimulate the amygdaloid nucleus
    B.	Stimulate a portion of the limbic system
    C.	Depress the hypothalamus
    D.	Depress the reticular system
    E.	All of the above Ref. 518 - p. 431

1188.	REGARDING THE ADMINISTRATION OF ANTIPSYCHOTIC DRUGS, IT HAS BEEN FOUND THAT:
    A.	Drugs administered intravenouly are three to four times more potent than given orally
    B.	Extended release capsules are desirable when high plasma levels are required
    C.	The enanthate ester is useful for intravenous preparations
    D.	Intravenous is preferable to intramuscular administration because painful areas of induration can be avoided
    E.	Urine tests for phenothiazine metabolites in the urine are most useful with "low-dose" drugs Ref. 518 - p. 435

1189.	A COMPLICATION OF PHENOTHIAZINE MEDICATION USUALLY OCCURRING LATE IN THE COURSE OF TREATMENT IS:
    A.	Cholestatic jaundice
    B.	Agranulocytosis
    C.	Eosinophilia
    D.	Dermatosis
    E.	Corneal and lens deposits Ref. 518 - p. 442

1190. ANTIPARKINSON AGENTS ADMINISTERED WITH PHENOTHIAZINES:
   A. Should be used routinely to avoid extrapyramidal syndromes that develop in the majority of patients
   B. May be cut suddenly as withdrawal effects do not develop to these agents
   C. Alleviate the mental confusion, dry mouth, blurred vision, and paralysis of bladder or bowel that may occur with phenothiazines
   D. All of the above
   E. None of the above   Ref. 518 - p. 443

1191. A COMPLICATION OF ANTIPSYCHOTIC DRUGS WHICH SHOWS A STEADY DECLINE IN PREVALENCE IS:
   A. Cholestatic jaundice
   B. Agranulocytosis
   C. Sudden, unexpected death
   D. Melanin deposits in the skin
   E. Corneal and lenticular deposits   Ref. 518 - p. 444

1192. GLUTETHIMIDE IS A DANGEROUS DRUG IN THAT:
   A. Very small overdoses can have a lethal effect
   B. It has a high potential for causing dependence
   C. It is unique among centrally acting depressants in having to be completely metabolized, and once in the body in being extremely hard to remove
   D. All of the above
   E. None of the above   Ref. 518 - p. 448

1193. THE POTENTIAL FOR ELICITING WITHDRAWAL SYNDROMES, BY ABUSE OF RELATIVELY LOWER MULTIPLES OF THE USUAL DAILY DOSE, IS HIGHEST WITH:
   A. Chlordiazepoxide
   B. Diazepam
   C. Short-acting barbiturates
   D. Moderately long-acting barbiturates
   E. Meprobamate   Ref. 518 - p. 450

1194. TRICYCLIC ANTIDEPRESSANTS DIFFER FROM PHENOTHIAZINES AND THIOXANTHENE ANTIPSYCHOTIC DRUGS IN THAT THEY:
   A. Facilitate adrenergic transmission
   B. Have less anticholinergic effect
   C. Do not cause EEG abnormalities
   D. Do not cause cholestatic jaundice
   E. Do not cause peripheral neuropathy
                                           Ref. 518 - p. 451

1195. ACCORDING TO FREUD, THE MOST IMPORTANT EVENT OF A MAN'S LIFE IS:
   A. The death of his mother
   B. The death of his father
   C. His marriage
   D. The birth of his first child
   E. None of the above   Ref. 519 - p. 26

1196. IN THE PROCESS OF TRANSFORMING THE LATENT THOUGHTS INTO
THE MANIFEST CONTENT OF A DREAM THE FACTOR AT WORK IS:
   A. Condensation
   B. Displacement
   C. Representability in visual images
   D. Secondary revision
   E. All of the above   Ref. 519 - pp. 379, 530

1197. PHENOMENA ASSOCIATED WITH LSD BUT NOT WITH CANNABIS
INCLUDE:
   A. Depersonalization
   B. Visual hallucinations
   C. Paranoid reactions
   D. Anxiety
   E. None of the above   Ref. 520 - p. 496

1198. PHYSICAL SIGNS AND SYMPTOMS FOUND IN CANNABIS INTOXICATION
INCLUDE THE FOLLOWING, EXCEPT:
   A. Pupillary constriction
   B. Conjunctival injection
   C. Hunger
   D. Thirst
   E. Increased frequency of urination
                              Ref. 520 - p. 496

1199.

   A. Should not be given in doses exceeding 800mg per day
   B. Has a relatively high milligram per milligram potency
   C. Is marketed for intravenous use
   D. Is the treatment of choice for delirium tremens
   E. None of the above   Ref. 521 - p. 44

1200.

A. Is an ineffective antipsychotic agent
B. Is an effective antidepressant
C. Was the first drug of its class to be tested in psychiatry
D. Produces less sedation than amitriptyline
E. All of the above   Ref. 521 - p. 12

1. Tecce, J.J.: Contingent Negative Variation and Individual Differences, Arch Gen Psychiat 24: 1-16, 1971

2. Smith, D.E. and Wesson, D.R.: Phenobarbital Technique for Treatment of Barbiturate Dependence, Arch Gen Psychiat 24: 56-60, 1971

3. Marmor, J.: Dynamic Psychotherapy and Behavior Therapy, Arch Gen Psychiat 24: 22-28, 1971

4. O'Brien, C.R., DiGiacomo, J.N., Fahn, S. and Schwartz, G.A.: Mental Effects of High Dosage Levodopa, Arch Gen Psychiat 24: 61-64, 1971

5. Wyatt, R.J., Portnoy, B., Kupfer, D.J., Snyder, F. and Engelman,K.: Resting Plasma Catecholamine Concentrations in Patients With Depression and Anxiety, Arch Gen Psychiat 24: 65-70, 1971

6. Jones, B.and Parsons, O.A.: Impaired Abstracting Ability in Chronic Alcoholics, Arch Gen Psychiat 24: 71-75, 1971

7. Goodwin, D.W., Alderson, P. and Rosenthal, R.: Clinical Significance of Hallucinations in Psychiatric Disorders, Arch Gen Psychiat 24: 76-80, 1971

8. Greenblatt, D.J. and Shader, R.I.: Meprobamate: A Study of Irrational Drug Use, Am J Psychiat 127: 1297-1303, 1971

9. Dohrenwend, B.P., Egri, G., Mendelsohn, E.S.: Psychiatric Disorder in General Populations: A Study of the Problem of Clinical Judgement, Am J Psychiat 127: 1304-1312, 1971

10. McKinney, W.T., Suomi, S.J., Harlow, H.F.: Depression in Primates, Am J Psychiat 127: 1313-1319, 1971

11. Ananth, J.V., Ban, T.A., Lehman, H.E., Rizvi, F.A.: An Adverse Reaction Unit, Results and Functions, Am J Psychiat 1339-1344, 1971

12. Darley, P.J. and Kenny, W.T.: Community Care and the "Queequeg Syndrome": A Phenomenological Evaluation of Methods of Rehabilitation for Psychotic Patients, Am J Psychiat 127: 1333-1338, 1971

13. Nelson, S.H. and Grunebaum, H.: A Follow-Up Study of Wrist Slashers, Am J Psychiat 127: 1345-1349, 1971

14. Kramer, M., Winget, C., Whitman, R.M.: A City Dreams: A Survey Approach to Normative Dream Content, Am J. Psychiat 127: 1350-1356, 1971

15. Herz, M.I., Endicott, J., Spitzer, R.I. and Mesnikoff, A.: Day Versus Inpatient Hospitalization, Am J Psychiat 127: 1371-1382, 1971

16. Zall, H.: Lithium Carbonate and Isocarboxazide: An Effective Drug Approach In Severe Depressions, Am J Psychiat 127: 1400-1403, 1971

17. Crane, G.E.: Persistence of Neurological Symptoms Due to Neuroleptic Drugs, Am J. Psychiat 127: 1407-1410, 1971

18. Wender, P.H., Epstein, R.S., Kopin, I.J. and Gordon, E.K.: Urinary
     Monoamine Metabolites In Children With Minimal Brain Dysfunction, Am J
     Psychiat 127: 1411-1415, 1971

19. Kubie, L.S.: The Retreat From Patients, Arch Gen Psychiat 24: 98-106, 1971

20. Vaillant, G.: Theoretical Hierarchy of Adaptive Ego Mechanisms, Arch Gen
     Psychiat 24: 107-118, 1971

21. Wyatt, R.J., Fram, D.H., Kupfer, D.J. and Snyder, F.: Total Prolonged
     Drug-Induced REM Sleep Suppression in Anxious-Depressed Patients,
     Arch Gen Psychiat 24: 145-155, 1971

22. Dorzab, J., Baker, M., Cadoret, R.J. and Winokur, G.: Depressive
     Disease: Familial Psychiatric Illness, Am J Psychiat 127: 1128-1133, 1971

23. Mirin, S.M., Shapiro, L.M., Meyer, R.E., Pillard, R.C., Fisher, S.:
     Casual Versus Heavy Use of Marijuana, Am J Psychiat 127: 1134-1139, 1971

24. Ellinwood, E.H.: Assault and Homicide Associated with Amphetamine Abuse,
     Am J Psychiat 127: 1170-1175, 1971

25. Muslin, H.L.: On Acquiring a Kidney, Am J Psychiat 127: 1185-1188, 1971

26. Abram, H.S., Moore, G.L. and Westerveslt, F.B.: Suicidal Behavior in
     Chronic Dialysis Patients, Am J Psychiat 127: 1199-1204, 1971

27. Bukatman, B.A., Foy, J.L. and Degrazia, E.: What is Competence
     Stand Trial?, Am J Psychiat 127: 1225-1229, 1971

28. Brown, E. and Barglow, P.: Pseudocyesis, Arch Gen Psychiat 24:
     221-229, 1971

29. Beigel, A. and Murphy, D.L.: Unipolar and Bipolar Affective Illness,
     Arch Gen Psychiat 24: 215-220, 1971

30. Durham, H.W.: Socio cultural Studies of Schizophrenia, Arch Gen Psychiat
     24: 206-214, 1971

31. Beiser, M.: A Study of Personality Assets in a Rural Community, Arch Gen
     Psychiat 24: 244-254, 1971

32. Litvak, R. and Kaelbing, R.: Agranulocytosis, Leukopenia, and Psychotropic
     Drugs, Arch Gen Psychiat 24: 265-267, 1971

33. Rothenberg, A.: The Process of Janusian Thinking in Creativity, Arch Gen
     Psychiat 24: 195-205, 1971

34. Stoller, A.: The Term "Transvestism", Arch Gen Psychiat 24: 231-237, 1971

35. Gilmour, D.G., Bloom, A.D., Lele, K.P., Robbins, E.S. and Maximilian
     C.: Chromosomal Aberrations in Users of Psychoactive Drugs, Arch Gen
     Psychiat 24: 268-272, 1971

36.   Lifton, R. J.: Protean Man, Arch Gen Psychiat 24: 298-304, 1971

37.   Paul, M.I., Cramer, H. and Goodwin,F.K.: Urinary Cyclic AMP Excretion
       in Depression and Mania, Arch Gen Psychiat 24: 327-333, 1971

38.   Shobe, F. O. and Brion, P.: Long-term Prognosis in Manic Depressive
       Illness, Arch Gen Psychiat 24: 334-337, 1971

39.   Hartmann, E., Baekeland, F., Zwilling, G. and Hoy, P.: Sleep Need:
       How Much Sleep and What Kind?, Am J Psychiat 127: 1001-1008, 1971

40.   Schildkraut, J. J., Winokur, A., Draskoczy, P.R. and Hensle, J.H.:
       Changes in Norepinephrine Turnover in Rat Brain During Chronic
       Administration of Imipramine and Protiptyline: A Possible Explanation for
       the Delay in Onset of Clinical Antidepressant Effects, Am J Psychiat 127:
       1032-1039, 1971

41.   Crane, G.E., Johnson, A.W. and Buffaloe, W.J.: Long-Term Treatment
       with Neuroleptic Drugs and Eye Opacities, Am J. Psychiat 127:
       1045-1047, 1971

42.   Heiser, J. F. and Gillin, J. C.: The Reversal of Anticholinergic Drug-
       Induced Delirium and Coma with Physostigmine, Am J Psychiat 127:
       1050-1054, 1971

43.   Paulson, G.W.: Use of Pyridoxine in Chorea, Am J Psychiat 127:
       1091-1092, 1971

44.   Kubie, L. S.: The Destructive Potential of Humor in Psychotherapy,
       Am J Psychiat 127: 861-866, 1971

45.   Zetzel, E.R.: A Developmental Approach to the Borderline Patient,
       Am J Psychiat 127: 867-871, 1971

46.   Bunney, W.E., Brodie, H.K.H., Murphy, D.L. and Goodwin, F.K.:
       Studies of Alphamethyl-para-tyrosine, L-dopa, and L-tryptophan in
       Depression and Mania, Am J Psychiat 127: 872-881, 1971

47.   Duncan, J.W. and Duncan, G.M.: Murder in the Family: A Study of
       Some Homicidal Adolescents, Am J Psychiat 127: 1498-1502, 1971

48.   Hussain, M. Z.: Desensitization and Flooding (Implosion) in Treatment of
       Phobias, Am J Psychiat 127: 1509-1514, 1971

49.   Voth, A. C. and Voth, H. M.: Further Experimental Studies of Mental
       Patients Through the Autokinetic Phenomenon, Am J Psychiat 127:
       1515-1520, 1971

50.   Altshuler, K. Z.: Studies of the Deaf: Relevance to Psychiatric Theory,
       Am J Psychiat 127, 1521-1526, 1971

51.   Fitzgerald, R. G.: Visual Phenomenology with Recently Blind Adults,
       Am J Psychiat 127: 1537-1539, 1971

52.   Freeman, D.A.: Congenital and Perinatal Sensory Deprivation: Some Studies
       in Early Development, Am J Psychiat 127: 1539-1545, 1971

53.   Small, J.G., Small, I.F., Moore, D.F.: Experimental Withdrawal of
      Lithium in Recovered Manic-Depressive Patients: A Report of 5 Cases,
      Am J Psychiat 127: 1555-1558, 1971

54.   Murphy, D.L., Goodwin, F.K., Bunney, W.E.: Leukocytosis During
      Lithium Treatment, Am J Psychiat 127: 15559-1561, 1971

55.   Reinhardt, R.F.: The Outstanding Jet Pilot, Am J Psychiat 127: 732-736, 1970

56.   Bidder, T.G., Strain, J.J., Brunschwig, L.: Bilateral and Unilateral ECT:
      Follow-Up Study and Critique, Am J Psychiat 127: 737-745, 1970

57.   Rosen, D.H.: The Serious Suicide Attempt: Epidemiological and Follow-Up
      Study of 886 Patients, Am J Psychiat 127: 764-770, 1970

58.   Meltzer, H.Y. and Moline, R.: Muscle Abnormalities in Acute Psychoses,
      Arch Gen Psychiat 23: 481-491, 1970

59.   Meltzer, H.Y. and Engel, W.K.: Histochemical Abnormalities in Skeletal
      Muscle in Acutely Psychotic Patients, Arch Gen Psychiat 23: 492-502, 1970

60.   Friedman, A.J.: Hostility Factors and Clinical Improvement in Depressed
      Patients, Arch Gen Psychiat 23: 524-537, 1970

61.   Marks, I.M.: Agoraphobic Syndrome, Arch Gen Psychiat 23: 538-553, 1970

62.   Holden, J.M.C., Itil, T.M. and Hofstatter, L.: Prefrontal Lobotomy:
      Stepping Stone or Pitfall, Am J Psychiat 127: 591-598, 1970

63.   Stabenau, J.R., Creveling,C.R. and Daly, J.: The "Pink Spot", 3, 4-
      Dimethoxyphenylehylamine, Common Tea, and Schizophrenia, Am J
      Psychiat 127: 611-616, 1970

64.   Wikler, A., Dixon, J.F., Parker, J.B.: Brain Function in Problem
      Children and Controls: Psychometric, Neurological, and EEG Comparison,
      Am J Psychiat 127: 634-645, 1970

65.   Dizmag, L.H. and Cheatham, C.F.: The Lesch-Nyhan Syndrome, Am J
      Psychiat 127: 671-677, 1970

66.   Woody, G.E.: Visual Disturbances Experienced by Hallucinogenic Drug
      Abusers While Driving, Am J Psychiat 127: 683-687, 1970

67.   Prien, R.F., DeLong, S.L., Cole, J.O. and Levine, J.: Ocular Changes
      with Prolonged High Dose Chlorpromazine Therapy, Arch Gen Psychiat 23:
      464-468, 1970

68.   Hoffer, A. and Pollin, W.: Schizophrenia in the NAS-NRC Panel of 15,909
      Veteran Twin Pairs, Arch Gen Psychiat 23: 469-477, 1970

69.   Black, S., Owens, K.L. and Wolff, R.P.: Patterns of Drug Use: A Study
      of 5,482 Subjects, Am J Psychiat 127: 420-423, 1970

70.   Fleminger, J.J., Horne, D.J.L., Nair, N.P.V. and Nott, P.N.:
      Differential Effects of Unilateral and Bilateral ECT, Am J Psychiat 127:
      430:436, 1970

71.   Allen, M.G. and Pollin, W.: Schizophrenia in Twins and the Diffuse Ego
      Boundary Hypothesis, Am J Psychiat 127: 437-442, 1970

72.   Kane, F.J., Lipton, M.A., Krall, A.R. and Obrist, P.A.: Psychoendocrine
      Study of Oral Contraceptive Agents, Am J Psychiat 127: 443-450, 1970

73.   Aronoff, M.S. and Epstein, R.S.: Factors Associated with Poor Response
      to Lithium Carbonate: A Clinical Study, Am J Psychiat 127: 472-480, 1970

74.   McKenna, G., Engle, R.P., Brooks, H. and Dalen, J.: Cardiac Arrhythmias
      During EST: Significance, Prevention and Treatment, Am J Psychiat 127:
      530-533, 1970

75.   Weiss, G., Minde, K., Werry, J.S., Douglas, V. and Nemeth, E.: Studies
      on the Hyperactive Child, Arch Gen Psychiat 24: 409-414, 1971

76.   Mosher, L.R., Pollin, W. and Stabenau, J.R.: Identical Twins Discordant for
      Schizophrenia, Arch Gen Psychiat 24: 422-430, 1971

77.   Offord, D.R. and Cross, L.A.: Adult Schizophrenia with Scholastic
      Failure of Low IQ in Childhood, Arch Gen Psychiat 24: 431-436, 1971

78.   Pardes, H., Winston, A. and Paparnik,D.S.: Reexamination of the A-B
      Field Dependence Relationship, Arch Gen Psychiat 24: 465-467, 1971

79.   Hankoff, L.D., Rabiner, C.J. and Hervey, C.S.G.: Comparison of the
      Satellite Clinic and Hospital-Based Clinic, Arch Gen Psychiat 24: 474-478, 1971

80.   Sachar, E.J., Hellman, L., Fukushima, D.K. and Gallagher, T.F.:
      Cortisol Production in Depressive Illness, Arch Gen Psychiat 23: 289-298, 1970

81.   Heninger, G.R., Mueller, P.S.: Carbohydrate Metabolism in Mania, Arch
      Gen Psychiat 23: 310-318, 1970

82.   Wikler, A.: Clinical and Social Aspects of Marijuana Intoxication, Arch
      Gen Psychiat 23: 320-325, 1970

83.   Bellak, L., Hurvich, M., Gediman, H. and Crawford, P.: Study of the Ego
      Functions of the Schizophrenic Syndrome, Arch Gen Psychiat 23:
      1326-1336, 1970

84.   A Family View of Hysterical Psychosis, Am J Psychiat 127: 280-285, 1970

85.   Alpert, M. and Silvers, K.N.: Perceptual Characteristics Distinguishing
      Auditory Hallucinations in Schizophrenia and Acute Alcoholic Psychoses,
      Am J Psychiat 127: 298-302, 1970

86.   Murphy, D.C., Colburn, R.W., Davis, J.M. and Bunney, W.E.: Imipramine
      and Lithium Effects on Biogenic Amine Transport in Depressed and Manic-
      Depressive Patients, Am J Psychiat 127: 339-345, 1970

87.   Van der Velde, C.D.: Effectiveness of Lithium Carbonate in the Treatment
      of Manic-Depressive Illness, Am J Psychiat 127: 345-351, 1970

88.   Platman, S.R.: A Comparison of Lithium Carbonate and Chlorpromazine
      in Mania, Am J Psychiat 127: 351-353, 1970

89.   McCabe, M.S., Reich, T. and Winokur, G.: Methysergide as a Treatment
      for Mania, Am J Psychiat 127: 354-356, 1970

90.   Bunney, W.E.: Present Status of Psychological Reactions to L-Dopa,
      Am J Psychiat 127: 361-362, 1970

91.   Schildkraut, J.J.: Neurochemical Studies of the Affective Disorders: The
      Pharmacological Bridge, Am J Psychiat 127: 358-360, 1970

92.   Clark, L.D., Hughes, R. and Nakashima, E.N.: Behavioral Effects of
      Marijuana, Arch Gen Psychiat 23: 193-198, 1970

93.   Melges, F.T., Tinklenberg, J.R., Hollister, L.E. and Gillespie, H.K.:
      Temporal Disintegration and Depersonalization During Marijuana Intoxica-
      tion, Arch Gen Psychiat 23: 204-210, 1970

94.   Kales, A., Preston, T.A., Tan, T.L. and Allen, C.: Hypnotics and
      Altered Sleep-Dream Patterns, Arch Gen Psychiat 23: 211-218, 1970

95.   Kales, A., Kales, J.D., Scharf, M.B. and Tan, T.L.: All Night EEG
      Studies of Chloral Hydrate, Flurazepam, and Methaqualone, Arch Gen
      Psychiat 23: 219-225, 1970

96.   Hollister, L.E.: Choice of Antipsychotic Drugs, Am J Psychiat 127:
      186-190, 1970

97.   Prange, A.J., Wilson, I.C., Knox, A., McClane, T.K. and Lipton, M.A.:
      Enhancement of Imipramine by Thyroid Stimulating Hormone: Clinical
      and Theoretical Implications, Am J Psychiat 127: 191-199, 1970

98.   Snyder, S.H., Taylor, K.M., Coyle, J.T. and Meyerhoff, J.L.: The
      Role of Brain Dopamine in Behavioral Regulation and the Action of
      Psychotropic Drugs, Am J Psychiat 127: 199-207, 1970

99.   Newman, L.E.: Transsexualism in Adolescence, Arch Gen Psychiat 23:
      112-121, 1970

100. Motto, J.A.: Newspaper Influence on Suicide, Arch Gen Psychiat 23:
      143-148, 1970

101. Attkisson, C.C.: Suicide in San Francisco Skid Row, Arch Gen Psychiat 23:
      149-157, 1970

102. Yufit, R.I., Benzies, B., Fante, M.E., Fawcett, J.A.: Suicide Potential
      and Time Perspective, Arch Gen Psychiat 23: 158-153, 1970

103. Kinzel, A.F.: Body-Buffer Zone in Violent Prisoners, Am J Psychiat 127:
      59-64, 1970

104. Jackson, B.: The Revised Diagnostic and Statistical Manual of the American
      Psychiatric Association, Am J Psychiat 127: 65-73, 1970

105. Knoff, W.F.: A History of the Concept of Neurosis, with a Memoir of
      William Cullen, Am J Psychiat 127: 80-84, 1970

106. Greenbaum, G. H.: An Evaluation of Niacinamide in the Treatment of
     Childhood Schizophrenia, Am J Psychiat 127: 89-92, 1970

107. Werble, B.: Second Follow-Up Study of Borderline Patients, Arch Gen
     Psychiat 23: 3-7, 1970

108. Poznanski, E. and Zrull, J. P.: Childhood Depression, Arch Gen Psychiat
     23: 8-15, 1970

109. Kahana, E. and Kahana, B.: Therapeutic Potential of Age Integration,
     Arch Gen Psychiat 23: 20-29, 1970

110. Kupfer, D. J., Wyatt, R. J., Greenspan, K. and Snyder, F.: Lithium
     Carbonate and Sleep in Affective Illness, Arch Gen Psychiat 23: 35-40, 1970

111. Spitzer, R. L., Endicott, J., Fleiss, J. L. and Cohen, J.: The Psychiatric
     Status Schedule, Arch Gen Psychiat 23: 41-55, 1970

112. Tkach, J. R. and Hokama, Y.: Autoimmunity in Chronic Brain Syndrome,
     Arch Gen Psychiat 23: 61-64, 1970

113. Zelman, J. and Guillan, R.: Heat Stroke in Phenothiazine-Treated Patients:
     A Report of Three Fatalities, Am J Psychiat 126: 1787-1790, 1970

114. Robbens, E. S., Robbens, L., Frosch, W. A. and Stern, M.: College Student
     Drug Use, Am J Psychiat 126: 1743-1751, 1970

115. Miller, P. R.: Social Activists and Social Change: The Chicago Demonstators,
     Am J Psychiat 126: 1752-1759, 1970

116. Tamerin, J. S., Weiner, S., Menderson, J.: Alcoholics' Expectancies and
     Recall of Experiences During Intoxication, Am J Psychiat 126: 1697-1704,
     1970

117. Leopold, R. J. and Kissich, W. L.: A Community Mental Health Center,
     Regional Medical Program and Joint Planning, Am J Psychiat 126 :
     1718-1726, 1970

118. Evans, J. L.: The College Student in the Psychiatric Clinic: Syndromes and
     Subcultural Sanctions, Am J Psychiat 126: 1736-1742, 1970

119. Stein, M.: Psychiatrist's Role in Psychiatric Research, Arch Gen Psychiat
     22: 481-489, 1970

120. Caldwell, D. F., Brane, A. J., Beckett, P. G. S.: Sleep Patterns in Normal
     and Psychotic Children, Arch Gen Psychiat 22: 500-503, 1970

121. Stoller, R. J.: Pornography and Perversion, Arch Gen Psychiat 22:
     490-499, 1970

122. Riskin, J. and Faunce, E. E.: Family Interaction Scales: III. Discussion of
     Methodology and Substantive Findings, Arch Gen Psychiat 22: 527-537, 1970

123. Glassman, B. M. and Siegel, A.: Personality Correlates of Survival in a
     Long Term Hemodialysis Program, Arch Gen Psychiat 22: 566-674, 1970

124.   Nicholi, A. M.: The Motorcycle Syndrome, Am J Psychiat 126: 1588-1595, 1970

125.   Green, R.: Persons Seeking Sex Change: Psychiatric Management of Special Problems, Am J Psychiat 126: 1596-1603, 1970

126.   Taintor, Z.: Birth Order and Psychiatric Problems in Boot Camp, Am J Psychiat 126: 1604-1610, 1970

127.   Zuithoff, D.: Community Psychiatry and Social Action - A Survey, Am J Psychiat 126: 1621-1627, 1970

128.   Satloff, A. and Worby, C. M.: The Psychiatric Emergency Service: Mirror of Change, Am J Psychiat 126: 1628-1632, 1970

129.   Rosenbaum, M. and Richman, J.: Suicide: The Role of Hostility and Death Wishes from the Family and Significant Others, Am J Psychiat 126: 1652-1655, 1970

130.   Cancro, R.: A Classificatory Principle in Schizophrenia, Am J Psychiat 126: 1655-1659, 1970

131.   Clark, G. R., Telfer, M. A., Baker, D., Rosen, M.: Sex Chromosomes, Crime and Psychosis, Am J Psychiat 126: 1659-1663, 1970

132.   Earle, B. V.: Thyroid Hormone and Tricyclic Antidepressants in Resistant Depressions, Am J Psychiat 126: 1667-1669, 1970

133.   Perkins, M. E. and Bloch, H. I.: Survey of a Methadone Maintenance Treatment Program, Am J Psychiat 126: 1289-1396, 1970

134.   Chatel, J. C. and Peele, R.: A Centennial Review of Neurasthenia, Am J Psychiat 126: 1389-1396, 1970

135.   Resnick, P.: Murder of the Newborn: A Psychiatric Review of Neonaticide, Am J Psychiat 126: 1414-1420, 1970

136.   Waggoner, R.: Restructuring the American Psychiatric Association for the 1970's, Am J Psychiat 126: 1490-1492, 1970

137.   Christmas, J. J., Wallace, H., Edwards, J.: New Careers and New Mental Health Services: Fantasy or Future, Am J Psychiat 126: 1480-1486, 1970

138.   Newman, L. E. and Steinberg, J. C.: Consultation with Police on Human Relations Training, Am J Psychiat 126: 1421-1429, 1970

139.   Kluger, J.: The Uninsulated Caseload in a Neighborhood Mental Health Center, Am J Psychiat 126, 1430-1436, 1970

140.   Fishman, J. R. and McCormack, J.: "Mental Health Without Walls": Community Mental Health in the Ghetto, Am J Psychiat 126: 1461-1467, 1970

141.   Lynch, M. and Gardner, E. A.: Some Issues Raised in the Training of Para-professional Personnel as Clinical Therapists, Am J Psychiat 126: 1473-1479, 1970

142.   Paul, M.I., Ditzion, B.R., Pauk, G.L. and Janowsky, D.S.: Urinary
       Adenosine 3',5'- Monophosphate Excretion in Affective Disorder, Am J
       Psychiat 126: 1493-1497, 1970

143.   Jansen, E.: The Role of the Halfway House in Community Mental Health
       Programs in the United Kingdom and America, Am J. Psychiat 126:
       1498-1504, 1970

144.   Jacobs, T.J. and Charles, E.: Correlation of Psychiatric Symptomatology
       and the Menstrual Cycle in an Outpatient Population, Am J Psychiat 126:
       1504-1508, 1970

145.   Shurley, J.T., Pierce, C.M., Natani, K. and Brooks, R.E.: Sleep
       and Activity Patterns at South Pole Station, Arch Gen Psychiat 22:
       385-389, 1970

146.   Meltzer, H.Y. and Moline, R.: Plasma Enzymatic Activity After Exercise,
       Arch Gen Psychiat 22: 390-397, 1970

147.   Meltzer, H.Y., Kupfer, D.J., Wyatt, R. and Snyder, F.: Sleep Disturbance
       and Serum CPK Activity in Acute Psychosis, Arch Gen Psychiat 22:
       398-405, 1970

148.   Johnson, L.C., Burdick, J.A. and Smith, J.: Sleep During Alcohol Intake
       and Withdrawal in the Chronic Alcoholic, Arch Gen Psychiat 22: 406-418,
       1970

149.   Nathan, P.E., Titler, N.A., Lowenstein, L.M., Solomon, P. and Rossi,
       A.M.: Behavioral Analysis of Chronic Alcoholism, Arch Gen Psychiat 22:
       419-430, 1970

150.   Treffert, D.A.: Epidemiology of Infantile Autism, Arch Gen Psychiat 22:
       431-438, 1970

151.   Hollander, M.H.: The Need or Wish to be Held, Arch Gen Psychiat 22:
       445-453, 1970

152.   Wang, H.S., Obrist, W.D., Busse, E.W.: Neurophysiological Correlates
       of the Intellectual Function of Elderly Persons Living in the Community,
       Am J Psychiat 126: 1205-1212, 1970

153.   Kupfer, D.J., Wyatt, R.J. Scott, J., Snyder, F.: Sleep Disturbances in
       Acute Schizophrenic Patients, Am J Psychiat 126: 1213-1223, 1970

154.   Whittington, H.G.: Evaluation of Therapeutic Abortion as an Element of
       Preventive Psychiatry, Am J Psychiat 126: 1224-1229, 1970

155.   Marder, L.: Psychiatric Experience with a Liberalized Abortion Law,
       Am J Psychiat 126: 1230-1236, 1970

156.   Klagsbrun, S.G.: Cancer, Emotions and Nurses, Am J Psychiat 126:
       1237-1243, 1970

157.   Fellner, C.H. and Marshall, J.R.: Kidney Donors - The Myth of Informed
       Consent, Am J Psychiat 126: 1245-1251, 1970

158.   Martin, C. C.: The Uniform Anatomical Gift Act, Am J Psychiat 126: 1252-1255, 1970

159.   Resnick, R. B., Fink, M., Freedman, A. M.: A Cyclazocine Typology in Opiate Dependence, Am J Psychiat 126: 1256-1260, 1970

160.   Brazelton, T. B.: Effect of Prenatal Drugs on the Behavior of the Neonate, Am J Psychiat 126: 1267-1274, 1970

161.   Biegel, A. and Feder, S. L.: Patterns of Utilization in Partial Hospitalization, Am J Psychiat 126: 1267-1274, 1970

162.   Ullman, M. and Krippner, S.: An Experimental Approach to Dreams and Telepathy: III. Report of Three Studies, Am J Psychiat 126: 1282-1289, 1970

163.   Mosher, L. R.: Nicotinic Acid Side Effects and Toxicity: A Review, Am J Psychiat 126: 1290-1296, 1970

164.   Angrist, B. M., Schweitzer, J. W., Gershon, S. Friedhoff, A. J.: Mephentermine Psychosis: Misuse of the Wyamine Inhaler, Am J Psychiat 126: 1315-1317, 1970

165.   Stroebel, C. F. and Glueck, B. C.: Computer Derived Global Judgments in Psychiatry, Am J Psychiat 126: 1057-1066, 1970

166.   Sacher, E. J., Kanter, S. S., Buie, D., Engle, R., Mehlman, R.: Psychoendocrinology of Ego Disintegration, Am J Psychiat 126: 1067-1078, 1970

167.   Blinder, B. J., Freeman, D. M. A., Stunkard, A. J.: Behavior Therapy of Anorexia Nervosa: Effectiveness of Activity as a Reinforcer of Weight Gain, Am J Psychiat 126: 1093-1098, 1970

168.   Blumer, D.: Hypersexual Episodes in Temporal Lobe Epilepsy, Am J Psychiat 126: 1099-1106, 1970

169.   Romano, J.: The Teaching of Psychiatry to Medical Students: Past, Present and Future, Am J Psychiat 126: 1115-1126, 1970

170.   Kaplan, H. M. and Blain, D.: Organizational Obstacles to Change in a Large Mental Hospital, Am J Psychiat 126: 1107-1114, 1970

171.   Miller, M. H., Fey, W. F., Greenfield, N. S.: The Implications of Changing Medical Education for Psychiatric Training Institutes, Am J Psychiat 126: 1127-1131, 1970

172.   Kaufman, M. R.: Psychiatry and Medical Education from the Vantage Point of 45 Years, Am J Psychiat 126: 1155-1157, 1970

173.   Edwards, J. G.: The Koro Pattern of Depersonalization in an American Schizophrenic Patient, Am J Psychiat 126: 1171-1173, 1970

174.   Schildkraut, J. J.: Tranylcypromine: Effects on Norepinephrine Metabolism in Rat Brain, Am J Psychiat 126: 925-931, 1970

175.   Grotjahn, M.: Psychiatric Consultations for Psychiatrists, Am J Psychiat 126: 932-937, 1970

176. Sandifer, M.G., Hordern, A., Green, L.M.: The Psychiatric Interview: The Import of the First Three Minutes, Am J Psychiat 126: 968-972, 1970

177. Small, I.F., Small, J.G., Alig, V.B., Moore, D.F.: Passive-Aggressive Personality Disorder: A Search for a Syndrome, Am J Psychiat 126: 973-983, 1970

178. Donnelly, J., Rosenberg, M., Fleeson, W.P.: The Evolution of the Mental Status: Past and Future, Am J Psychiat 126: 997-1002, 1970

179. Kane, F.J.: Treatment of Mania with Cinanserin, an Antiserotonin Agent, Am J Psychiat 126: 1020-1023, 1970

180. Liddon, S.C.: Sleep Paralysis, Psychosis and Death, Am J Psychiat 126: 1027-1031, 1970

181. Iwai, H. and Reynolds, D.K.: Morita Psychotherapy: The View from the West, Am J Psychiat 126: 1031-1035, 1970

182. Curry, S.H., Marshall, J.H.L., Davis, J.M., Janowsky, D.S.: Chlorpromazine Plasma Levels and Effects, Arch Gen Psychiat 22: 289-296, 1970

183. Platman, S.R., Fieve, R.R., Pierson, R.N.: Effect of Mood and Lithium Carbonate on Total Body Potassium, Arch Gen Psychiat 22: 297-300, 1970

184. Kerry, R.J., Owen, G.: Lithium Carbonate as a Mood and Total Body Water Stabilizer, Arch Gen Psychiat 22: 301-303, 1970

185. Sacher, E.J., Hellman, L., Kream, L., Fukushima, D.K., Gallagher, T.: Effect of Lithium Carbonate Therapy on Adrenocortical Activity, Arch Gen Psychiat 22: 304-307, 1970

186. Stuen, M.R., Solberg, K.B.: Maximal Hospital Benefits vs. Against Medical Advice, Arch Gen Psychiat 22: 351-355, 1970

187. Marohn, R.C.: The Therapeutic Milieu as an Open System, Arch Gen Psychiat 22: 360-364, 1970

188. Baekeland, F.: Exercise Deprivation, Arch Gen Psychiat 22: 365-369, 1970

189. Fitzgerald, R.G.: Reactions to Blindness, Arch Gen Psychiat 22: 370-379, 1970

190. Callaway, E.: Schizophrenia and Interference, Arch Gen Psychiat 22: 193-208, 1970

191. Curry, S.H., Davis, J.M., Janowsky, D.S., Marshall, J.H.L.: Factors Affecting Chlorpromazine Levels in Psychiatric Patients, Arch Gen Psychiat 22: 209-215, 1970

192. Mueller, P.S., Davis, J.M., Bunney, W.E., Weil-Malherbe, H., Cardon, P.V.: Plasma Free Fatty Acids Concentrations in Depressive Illness, Arch Gen Psychiat 22: 216-221, 1970

193. King, L.J., Pittman, G.D.: A Six-Year Follow-Up Study of 65 Adolescent Patients, Arch Gen Psychiat 22: 230-236, 1970

194. Umphress, A., Murphy, S., Nickols, J., Hammar, S.: Adolescent Enuresis, Arch Gen Psychiat 22: 237-244, 1970

195. Giovacchini, P.L.: Characterological Problems: The Need to be Helped, Arch Gen Psychiat 22: 245-251, 1970

196. Janowsky, D.S., Leff, M., Epstein, R.S.: Playing the Manic Game, Arch Gen Psychiat 22: 252-261, 1970

197. Lipkin, K.M., Dyrud, J., Meyer, G.G.: The Many Faces of Mania, Arch Gen Psychiat 22: 262-267, 1970

198. Hirsch, J.G., Borowitz, G.H., Costello, J.: Individual Differences in Ghetto 4-Year-Olds, Arch Gen Psychiat 22: 268-276, 1970

199. Small, J.G.:Small Sharp Spikes in a Psychiatric Population, Arch Gen Psychiat 22: 277-284, 1970

200. Waskow, I.E., Olsson, J.E., Salzman, C., Katz, M.M.: Psychological Effects of Tetrahydrocannabinol, Arch Gen Psychiat 22: 97-107, 1970

201. Baer, L., Platman, S.R., Fieve, R.R.: The Role of Electrolytes in Affective Disorders, Arch Gen Psychiat 22: 108-113, 1970

202. Rochford, J.M., Detre, T., Tucker, G.J., Harrow, M.: Neuro-psychological Impairments in Functional Psychiatric Diseases, Arch Gen Psychiat 22: 114-119, 1970

203. Kramer, M.: Manifest Dream Content in Normal and Psychopathologic States, Arch Gen Psychiat 22: 149-159, 1970

204. Siegel, A.: A Hospital Program for Young Adolescents, Arch Gen Psychiat 22: 166-178, 1970

205. Smith, B.M., Hain, J.D., Stevenson, I.: Controlled Interviews Using Drugs, Arch Gen Psychiat 22: 2-10, 1970

206. Paykel, E.S., Klerman, G.L., Prusoff, B.A.: Treatment Setting and Clinical Depression, Arch Gen Psychiat 22: 11-21, 1970

207. Fiske, D.W., Hunt, H.F., Luborsky, L., Orne, M.T., Parloff, M.B., Reiser, M.F., Tuma, A.H.: Planning of Research on Effectiveness of Psychotherapy, Arch Gen Psychiat 22: 22-32, 1970

208. Freedman, A., Luborsky, L., Harvey, R.B.: Dream Time (REM) and Psychotherapy, Arch Gen Psychiat 22: 33-39, 1970

209. Baer, L., Durell, J., Bunney, W.E., Levy, B.S., Murphy, D.L., Greenspan, K., Cardon, P.V.: Sodium Balance and Distribution in Lithium Carbonate Therapy, Arch Gen Psychiat 22: 63-71, 1970

210. Vandersale, T.A., Wiener, J.M.: Children Who Set Fires, Arch Gen Psychiat 22: 63-71, 1970

211. Baldessarini, R.J., Stephens, J.H.: Lithium Carbonate for Affective Disorders, Arch Gen Psychiat 22: 72-77, 1970

212. Chodoff, P.: The German Concentration Camp as a Psychological Stress,
      Arch Gen Psychiat 22: 78-87, 1970

213. Calef, V.: On the Current Concept of the Transference Neurosis,
      J Am Psa Assn 19: 22-25, 1971

214. Blum, H.P.: On the Conception and Development of the Transference
      Neurosis, J Am Psa Assn 19: 41-53, 1971

215. Weinshel, E.M.: The Transference Neurosis: A Survey of the Literature,
      J Am Psa Assn 19: 67-87, 1971

216. Stromgren, E.: Uses and Abuses of Concepts in Psychiatry,
      Am J Psychiat 126: 777-788, 1969

217. Rada, R.T., Daniels, R.S., Draper, E.: An Outpatient Setting for Treating
      Clinically Ill Psychiatric Patients, Am J Psychiat 126: 789-795, 1969

218. DiMascio, A. and Shader, R.I.: Drug Administration Schedules,
      A, J Psychiat 126: 796-801, 1969

219. Comer, J.P.: White Racism: Its Root, Form, and Foundation
      Am J Psychiat 126: 802-806, 1969

220. Crancer, A. and Quiring, D.L.: The Mentally Ill as Motor Vehicle Operator,
      Am J Psychiat 126: 807-813, 1969

221. Swanson, D.W. and Stipes, A.H.: Psychiatric Aspects of Klinefelter's
      Syndrome, Am J Psychiat 126: 814-822, 1969

222. Gottschalk, L.A. and Pattison, E.M.: Psychiatric Perspectives on T Groups
      and the Laboratory Movement, Am J Psychiat 126: 823-839, 1969

223. Kuehn, J.L. and Crinella, F.M.: Sensitivity Training: Interpersonal
      "Overkill" and Other Problems, Am J Psychiat 126:840-845, 1969

224. Hanson, P.G., Rothaus, P., O'Connell, W.E., Wiggens, G.: Training
      Patients for Effective Participation in Back-Home Groups,
      Am J Psychiat 126: 857-862, 1969

225. Crawshaw, R.: How Sensitive is Sensitivity Training?,
      Am J Psychiat, 126: 868-873, 1969

226. deMarneffe, F.: The New APA Standards for Psychiatric Facilities,
      Am J Psychiat, 126: 879-881, 1969

227. Mora, G.: 1969 Anniversaries, Am J Psychiat, 126: 892-897, 1969

228. Nussbaum, K., Schneidmuhl, A.M., Shaffer, J.W.: Psychiatric Assess-
      ment in the Social Security Program of Disability Insurance,
      Am J Psychiat 126: 879-881, 1969

229. Pollin, W., Allen, M.G., Hoffer, A., Stabenau, J.R., Hrubec, Z.:
      Psychopathology in 15,909 Pairs of Veteran Twins: Evidence for a Genetic
      Factor in the Pathogenesis of Schizophrenia and Its Relative Absence in
      Psychoneurosis, Am J Psychiat 126: 597-610, 1969

230. Judd, L.L., Brandkamp, W.W., McGlothlin, W.H.: Comparison of the Chromosomal Patterns Obtained from Groups of Continued Users, Former Users, and Nonusers of LSD-25, Am J Psychiat 126: 626-635, 1969

231. Gardner, R.A.: The Guilt Reaction of Parents of Children with Severe Physical Disease, Am J Psychiat 126: 636-644, 1969

232. Avnet, H.H.: Psychiatric Insurance - Ten Years Later, Am J Psychiat 126: 667-674, 1969

233. Glasser, M.A., Duggan, T.: Prepaid Psychiatric Care Experience with UAW Members, Am J Psychiat 126: 675-681, 1969

234. Green, E.L.: Psychiatric Services in a California Group Health Plan, Am J Psychiat 126: 681-688, 1969

235. Weinberg, J.: Sexual Expression in Later Life, Am J Psychiat 126: 713-716, 1969

236. Kaufman, J., Allen, J.R., West, L.J.: Runaways, Hippies, and Marijuana, Am J Psychiat 126: 717-720, 1969

237. Prange, A.J., Wilson, I.C., Rabon, A.M., Lipton, M.A.: Enhancement of Imipramine Antidepressant Activity by Thyroid Hormone, Am J Psychiat 126: 457-469, 1969

238. Babiyian, H.M., Odoroff, C.L.: The Mortality Experience of a Population With Psychiatric Illness, Am J Psychiat 126: 470-480, 1969

239. Johnson, F.G.: LSD in the Treatment of Alcoholism, Am J Psychiat 126: 481-487, 1969

240. Kollar, E.J., Pasnau, R.O., Rubin, R.T., Naitoh, P., Slater, G.G., Kales, A.: Psychological, Psychophysiological, and Biochemical Correlates of Prolonged Sleep Deprivation, Am J Psychiat 126: 488-497, 1969

241. Stephens, J.H., O'Conner, G., Wiener, G.: Long Term Prognosis in Schizophrenia Using the Becher-Wittner Scale, Am J Psychiat 126: 498-504, 1969

242. Mannino, F.V., Delgado, R.A.: Trichotillomania in Children: A Review, Am J Psychiat 126: 505-511, 1969

243. Robez, A., Bogard, W.J.:The Compleat Forensic Psychiatrist, Am J Psychiat 126: 519-525, 1969

244. Bartner, J.T., Reite, M.: Crime and LSD: The Insanity Plea, Am J Psychiat 126: 531-537, 1969

245. Greenland, C.: Appealing Against Commitment to Mental Hospitals in the UK, Canada, and the US, Am J Psychiat 126: 538-542, 1969

246. Modlen, H.C.: Psychiatry and the Courts: Some Promising Approaches, Am J Psychiat 126: 547-548, 1969

247. Whitten, J.R.: Psychical Seizures, Am J Psychiat 126: 560-565, 1969

248.   Horowitz, M.J.: Flashbacks: Recurrent Intrusive Images After the Use of LSD, Am J Psychiat 126: 565-569, 1969

249.   Hussar, A.E., Bragg, D.G.: The Effects of Chlorpromazine on the Swallowing Function in Chronic Schizophrenic Patients, Am J Psychiat 126: 570-573, 1969

250.   Allen, M.G., Pollin, W., Hoffer, A.: Parental, Birth, and Infancy Factors in Infant Twin Development, Am J Psychiat 127: 1597-1604, 1971

251.   Malitz, S., Kanzler, M.: Are Antidepressants Better Than Placebo?, Am J Psychiat 127 : 1605-1611, 1971

252.   Wharton, R.N., Perel, J.M., Dayton, P.G., Malitz, S.: A Potential Clinical Use for Methyphenidate with Tricyclic Antidepressants, Am J Psychiat 127: 1619-1625, 1971

253.   Penick, S.B., Buonpane, N., Carrier, R.N.: Short Term Acute Psychiatric Care: A Follow-Up Study, Am J Psychiat 127: 1626-1630, 1971

254.   Hildreth, A.M., Derogatis, L.R., McCusker, K.: Body Buffer Zone and Violence, Am J Psychiat 127: 1641-1645, 1971

255.   Weiner, S., Tamerin, J.S., Steinglass, P., Mendelson, J.H.: Familial Patterns in Chronic Alcoholism, Am J Psychiat 127: 1646-1653, 1971

256.   Tamerin, J.S., Weiner, S., Popper, R., Steinglass, P., Mendelson, J.H.: Alcohol and Memory, Am J Psychiat 127: 1659-1664, 1971

257.   Goodwin, D.W.: Two Species of Alcoholic "Blackout", Am J Psychiat 127: 1665-1670, 1971

258.   Bowers, M.B., Van Woert, M., Davis, L.: Sexual Behavior During L-Dopa Treatment for Parkinsonism, Am J Psychiat 127: 1691-1693, 1971

259.   Borge, G.F., Buchsbaum, M., Goodwin, F., Murphy, D., Silverman, J.: Neuropsychological Correlates of Affective Disorder, Arch Gen Psychiat 24: 501-508, 1971

260.   Schuckit, M., Robins, E., Feighner, J.: Tricyclic Antidepressants and MAO Inhibitors, Arch Gen Psychiat 24: 509-514, 1971

261.   Liberman, R.P.: Depression: A Behavioral Formulation, Arch Gen Psychiat 24: 515-523, 1971

262.   Robinson, D.S., Davis, J.M., Nies, A., Ravaris, C.L., Sylvester, D.: Relation of Sex and Aging to MAO Activity of the Human Brain, Plasma, and Platelets, Arch Gen Psychiat 24: 536-539, 1971

263.   Baekeland, F., Hay, P.: Reported vs. Recorded Sleep Characteristics, Arch Gen Psychiat 24: 548-551, 1971

264.   Korein, J., Fish, B., Shapiro, T., Gerner, E., Levidow, L.: EEG and Behavioral Effects of Drug Therapy in Children, Arch Gen Psychiat 24: 552-563, 1971

265.   Melges, F.T., Tinkelberg, J.R., Hollister, L.E., Gillespie, H.K.:
       Marijuana and the Temporal Span of Awareness,
       Arch Gen Psychiat 24: 564-567, 1971

266.   Meltzer, H.Y., Nankin, R., Raferty, J.: Serum Creatine Phosphokinase
       Activity in Newly Admitted Psychiatric Patients,
       Arch Gen Psychiat 24: 568-572, 1971

267.   Bloch, H.S.: Army Clinical Psychiatry in the Combat Zone - 1967-1968,
       Am J Psychiat 126: 289-298, 1969

268.   Friedman, H.J.: Some Problems of Inpatient Management with Borderline
       Patients, Am J Psychiat 126: 299-304, 1971

269.   Prien, R.F., Levine, J., Cole, J.O.: High Dose Trifluoperazine Therapy
       in Chronic Schizophrenia, Am J Psychiat 126: 305-313, 1969

270.   Murphy, G.E., Wetzel, R.D., Swallow, C.S., McClure, J.N.: Who Calls
       the Suicide Prevention Center, Am J Psychiat 126: 314-324, 1969

271.   Resnick, P.J.: Child Murder by the Parents: A Psychiatric Review of
       Filicide, Am J Psychiat 126: 325-334, 1969

272.   Balcanoff, E.J., McGarry, A.L.: Amicus Curiae: The Role of the Psychia-
       trist in Pretrial Examination, Am J Psychiat 126: 342-347, 1969

273.   Kimball, C.P.: Psychological Responses to the Experiences of Open
       Heart Surgery, Am J Psychiat 126: 348-359, 1969

274.   Rubinstein, D., Thomas, J.K.: Psychiatric Findings in Cardiotomy Patients,
       Am J Psychiat 126: 360-369, 1969

275.   Lunde, D.T.: Psychiatric Complications of Heart Transplant,
       Am J Psychiat 126: 369-373, 1969

276.   Eisendrath, R.M.,: The Role of Grief and Fear in the Death of Kidney
       Transplant Patients, Am J Psychiat 126: 381-387, 1969

277.   Morse, R.M., Litin, E.M.: Postoperative Delirium: A Study of Etiologic
       Factors, Am J Psychiat 126: 388-395, 1969

278.   Flor-Henry, P.: Schizophrenic-Like Reactive and Affective Psychoses
       Associated with Temporal Lobe Epilepsy: Etiologic Factors,
       Am J Psychiat 126: 400-404, 1969

279.   Silver, L.B., Dublin, C.C., Loerie, R.S.: Does Violence Breed Violence?,
       Am J Psychiat 126: 404-407, 1969

280.   Buchsbaum, M., Goodwin, F., Murphy, D., Borge, G.: AER in Affective
       Disorders, Am J Psychiat 128: 19-25, 1971

281.   Carpenter, W.T., Bunney, W.E.: Adrenal Cortical Activity in Depressive
       Illness, Am J Psychiat 128: 31-40, 1971

282.   Langenauer, B.S., Bowden, C.L.: A Follow-Up Study of Narcotic Addicts in
       the NARA Program, Am J Psychiat 128: 41-46, 1971

283. Seligman, R., MacMillan, B.G., Carroll, S.S.: The Burned Child: A Neglected Area of Psychiatry, Am J Psychiat 128: 52-57, 1971

284. Pasnau, R.O., Bayley, S.J.: Personality Changes in the First Year of Psychiatric Residence Training, Am J Psychiat 128: 79-84, 1971

285. Davies, R.K., Tucker, G.J., Harrow, M., Detre, T.P.: Confusional Episodes and Antidepressant Medication, Am J Psychiat 128:95-99, 1971

286. Demers, R.G., Heninger, G.R.: Sodium Intake and Lithium Treatment in Mania, Am J Psychiat 128: 100-104, 1971

287. Lipsitt, P.D., Lelos, D., McGarry, A.L.: Competancy for Trial: A Screening Instrument, Am J Psychiat 128: 105-109, 1971

288. Morse, R.M., Litin, R.M.: The Anatomy of a Delirium, Am J Psychiat 128: 111-116, 1971

289. Gershon, E.S., Dunner, D.L., Goodwin, K.T.: Toward a Biology of Affective Disorder, Arch Gen Psychiat 25: 1-15, 1971

290. Yalom, I.D., Liberman, M.A.: A Study of Encounter Group Casualties, Arch Gen Psychiat 25: 16-30, 1971

291. Derogatis, L.R., Cori, L., Lipman, R.S., Davis, D.M., Rickels, K.: Social Class and Race as Mediator Variables in Neurotic Symptomatology, Arch Gen Psychiat 25: 31-40, 1971

292. Fischer, A., Weinstein, M.R.: Mental Hospitals, Prestige, and the Image of Enlightenment, Arch Gen Psychiat 25: 41-48, 1971

293. Burnell, G.M.: Financing Mental Health Care, Arch Gen Psychiat 25: 49-55, 1971

294. Hauri, P., Hawkins, D.R.: Phasic REM, Depression, and the Relationship Between Sleeping and Waking, Arch Gen Psychiat 25: 56-63, 1971

295. Weiss, J.M., Kaufman, H.S.: A Subtle Organic Component in Some Cases of Mental Illness, Arch Gen Psychiat 25: 74-78, 1971

296. Moldofsky, H.: A Psychophysiological Study of Multiple Tics, Arch Gen Psychiat 28: 79-87, 1971

297. Rosenthal, A.J., Levine, S.U.: Brief Psychotherapy with Children, Am J Psychiat 128: 141-146, 1971

298. Liberman, R.P., Sonnenberg, S.M., Stern, M.S.: Psychiatric Evaluations for Young Men Facing the Draft, Am J Psychiat 128: 147-152, 1971

299. Rogers, M.P., Whybrow, P.C.: Clinical Hypothyroidism Occurring During Lithium Treatment, Am J Psychiat 128: 158-163, 1971

300. Jenkins, R.L.: The Runaway Reaction, Am J Psychiat 128: 168-173, 1971

301.   Steinberg, G. G., Troshinsky, C., Steinberg, H. R.: Dextroamphetamine-
       Responsive Behavior Disorder in School Children,
       Am J Psychiat 128: 174-179, 1971

302.   Saghir, M. T.: A Comparison of Some Aspects of Structured and Unstructured
       Psychiatric Interviews, Am J Psychiat 128: 180-184, 1971

303.   Danilowicz, D. A., Gabriel, H. P.: Postoperative Reactions in Children,
       Am J Psychiat 128: 185-188, 1971

304.   Secretary of Health, Education, and Welfare: Marijuana and Health:
       A Report to Congress (Summary), Am J Psychiat 128: 189-193, 1971

305.   Munoz, R. A., Marten, S., Gentry, K. A., Robins, E.: Mortality Following
       a Psychiatric Emergency Room Visit, Am J Psychiat 128: 220-224, 1971

306.   Garetz, C.: Group Rounds Versus Individual Medical Rounds on a Psychiatric
       In-Patient Service, Am J Psychiat 128: 227-229, 1971

307.   Dornbush, R. L., Fink, M., Freedman, A.: Marijuana, Memory, and
       Perception, Am J Psychiat 128: 194-197, 1971

308.   Meyer, R. E., Pillard, R. C., Shapiro, L. M., Mirin, S. M.: Administration
       of Marijuana to Heavy and Casual Marijuana Users,
       Am J Psychiat 128: 198-203, 1971

309.   Colbach, E.: Marijuana Use by GIs in Viet Nam,
       Am J Psychiat 128: 204-207, 1971

310.   Lipp, M., Benson, S. G., Taintor, Z.: Marijuana Use by Medical Students,
       Am J Psychiat 128: 207-212, 1971

311.   Keeler, M. H., Ewing, J. A., Rouse, B. A.: Hallucinogenic Effects of
       Marijuana as Currently Used, Am J Psychiat 128: 213-216, 1971

312.   Weissman, M. W., Klerman, G. L., Paykel, E. S.: Clinical Evaluation of
       Hostility in Depression, Am J Psychiat 128: 261-274, 1971

313.   McKegney, F. P., Lange, P.: The Decision to No Longer Live on Chronic
       Hemodialysis, Am J Psychiat 128: 267-274, 1971

314.   Steinglass, P., Weiner, S., Mendelson, J. H.: Interactional Issues as
       Determinants of Alcoholism, Am J Psychiat 128: 275-280, 1971

315.   Lorei, T. W., Gurel, L.: A Systematic Approach to Disposition Decisions,
       Am J Psychiat 128: 281-285, 1971

316.   Barcai, A.: Family Therapy in the Treatment of Anorexia Nervosa,
       Am J Psychiat 128: 286-290, 1971

317.   Hodges, E. F.: Crime Prevention by the Indeterminate Sentence Law,
       Am J Psychiat 128: 291-295, 1971

318.   Trinder, J., Kramer, M.: Dream Recall, Am J Psychiat 128: 296-301, 1971

319.   Kety, S.S., Rosenthal, D., Wender, P.H., Schulsinger, F.: Mental Illness
       in the Biological and Adoptive Families of Adopted Schizophrenics,
       Am J Psychiat 128: 302-306, 1971

320.   Rosenthal, D., Wender, P.H., Kety, S.S., Welner, J., Schulsinger, F.:
       The Adopted Away Offspring of Schizophrenics,
       Am J Psychiat 128: 307-311, 1971

321.   Pollin, W.: A Possible Genetic Factor Related to Psychosis,
       Am J Psychiat 128: 311-317, 1971

322.   Yarden, P.E., Discipio, W.J.: Abnormal Movements and Prognosis in
       Schizophrenia, Am J Psychiat 128: 317-323, 1971

323.   Jordan, K., Prugh, D.G.: Schizophreniform Psychosis of Childhood,
       Am J Psychiat 128: 328-331, 1971

324.   Ziskind, E., Somerfeld, E., Jens, R.: Can Schizophrenia Change to
       Affective Psychosis?, Am J Psychiat 128: 331-335, 1971

325.   Saletu, B., Itil, T.M., Saletu, M.: Auditory Evoked Response, EEG,
       and Thought Process in Schizophrenics, Am J Psychiat 128: 336-344, 1971

326.   Arieti, S.: Schizophrenia (Editorial), Am J Psychiat 128:348-350, 1971

327.   Muller, D.J.: ECT in LSD Psychosis, Am J Psychiat 128: 351-352, 1971

328.   Ziferstein, I.: Effects of Observation on the Therapeutic Process,
       Am J Psychiat 128: 353-355, 1971

329.   Wilkins, W.: Psychoanalytic and Behavioristic Approaches Toward
       Depression: A Synthesis?, Am J Psychiat 128: 358-359, 1971

330.   Bey, D.R., Smith, W.E.: Organizational Consultation in a Combat Unit,
       Am J Psychiat 128: 401-406, 1971

331.   Becker, A., Wylan, L., McCourt, W.: Primary Prevention - Whose
       Responsibility?, Am J Psychiat 128: 412-417, 1971

332.   Marohn, R.C., Offer, D., Ostrov, E.: Juvenile Delinquents View Their
       Impulsivity, Am J Psychiat 128: 418-423, 1971

333.   Menninger, W.W.: The Psychiatrist and the Violence Commission,
       Am J Psychiat 128: 431-436, 1971

334.   Gorney, R.: Interpersonal Intensity, Competition and Synergy,
       Am J Psychiat 128: 436-445, 1971

335.   Gardner, G.: Aggression and Violence - The Enemies of Precision
       Learning in Children, Am J Psychiat 128: 445-450, 1971

336.   Gault, W.B.: Some Remarks on Slaughter, Am J Psychiat 128:450-455, 1971

337.   Rothenberg, A.: On Anger, Am J Psychiat 128: 454-460, 1971

338.   Malmquist, C.P.: Premonitory Signs of Homicidal Aggression in
       Juveniles, Am J Psychiat 128: 461-465, 1971

339. Gottheil, E., Corbett, L.O., Grasberger, J.C., Cornelison, F.S.: Treating The Alcoholic in the Presence of Alcohol, Am J Psychiat 128: 475-480, 1971

340. Saraf, K., Klein, D.F.: The Safety of a Single Daily Dose Schedule for Imipramine, Am J Psychiat 128: 483-484, 1971

341. Stevens, H.: Gilles de la Tourette and his Syndrome by Serendipity, Am J Psychiat 128: 489-492, 1971

342. Raskin, D.E.: Problems in the Therapeutic Community, Am J Psychiat 128: 492-493, 1971

343. Davies, R.K., Detre, T.P., Egger, M.D., Tucker, G.J., Wyman, R.S.: Electroconvulsive Therapy Instruments, Arch Gen Psychiat 25: 97-99, 1971

344. Beresford, H.R.: Legal Issues Relating to Electroconvulsive Therapy, Arch Gen Psychiat 25: 100-102, 1971

345. Smith,W.G.: Critical Life Events and Prevention Strategies in Mental Health, Arch Gen Psychiat 25: 103-109, 1971

346. Kendall, R.E., Cooper, H.E., Gourlay, A.J., Copeland, H.R.M., Scharpe, L., Gurland, B.J.: Diagnostic Criteria of American and British Psychiatrists, Arch Gen Psychiat 25: 123-130, 1971

347. Lazare, A.: The Hysterical Character in Psychoanalytic Theory, Arch Gen Psychiat 25: 131-137, 1971

348. Fish, B.: The "One Child, One Drug" Myth of Stimulants in Hyper-Kinesis, Arch Gen Psychiat 25: 193–203, 1971

349. Gittelman-Klein, R., Klein, D.F.: Controlled Imipramine Treatment of School Phobia, Arch Gen Psychiat 25: 204-207, 1971

350. Kafka, J.S.: Ambiguity for Individuation, Arch Gen Psychiat 25: 232-239,1971

351. Fawcett, J.: Dextroamphetamine Response as a Possible Predictor of Improvement With Tricyclic Therapy in Depression, Arch Gen Psychiat 25: 247-255, 1971

352. Sachar, E.J., Finkelstein, J., Hellman, L.: Growth Hormone Responses in Depressive Illness, Arch Gen Psychiat 25: 263-269, 1971

353. Carpenter, W.T., Bunney, W.E.: Diurnal Rhythm of Cortisol in Mania, Arch Gen Psychiat 25: 270-273, 1971

354. Mendels, J., Hawkins, D.R.: Longitudinal Sleep in Hypomania, Arch Gen Psychiat 25: 274-277, 1971

355. Hughes, P., Chappel, J., Sencey, E., Jaffe, J.: Developing Inpatient Services for Community-Based Treatment of Narcotic Addiction, Arch Gen Psychiat 25 : 278-283, 1971

356. Lu, L., Stotsky, B.A., Cole, J.O.: A Controlled Study of Drugs in Long-term Geriatric Psychiatric Patients, Arch Gen Psychiat 25: 284-288, 1971

357. Panzetta, A. F.: The Concept of Community, Arch Gen Psychiat 25: 291-297, 1971

358. Dyrud, J.: Treatment of Anxiety States, Arch Gen Psychiat 25: 298-305, 1971

359. Chessick, R.D.: Use of the Couch in the Psychotherapy of Borderline Patients, Arch Gen Psychiat 25: 306-313, 1971

360. Birk, L., Huddleston, W., Miller, E., Cohler, B.: Avoidance Conditioning For Homosexuality, Arch Gen Psychiat 25: 314-323, 1971

361. Hillman, R.G.: The Teaching of Psychotherapy Problems by Computer, Arch Gen Psychiat 25: 324-329, 1971

362. Paykel, E.S., Prusoff, G.A., Uhlenhuth E.H.: Scaling of Life Events, Arch Gen Psychiat 25: 340-347, 1971

363. Dunner, D.L., Gershon, E.S., Goodwin, F.K.: Differential COMT Activity in Unipolar and Bipolar Affective Illness, Arch Gen Psychiat 25: 348-353, 1971

364. Papeschi, R., McClure,: HVA and 5-HIAA in CSF of Depressed Patients, Arch Gen Psychiat 25: 354-358, 1971

365. Benkert, O., Renz, A., Marano, C., Matussek, N.: Altered Tyrosine Daytime Levels in Endogenous Depressive Patients, Arch Gen Psychiat 25: 353-363, 1971

366. Dorus, E., Dorus, W., Rechtschaffen, A.: The Incidence of Novelty in Dreams, Arch Gen Psychiat 25: 364-368, 1971

367. Mellinger, G.D., Balter, M.B., Manheimer, D.I.: Patterns of Psychotherapeutic Drugs Among Adults in San Francisco, Arch Gen Psychiat 25: 385-394, 1971

368. Clark, M.C., Huber, W.K., Charalampous, K.D., Serafetinides, E.A., Trousdale, W., Colemore, J.P.: Drug Treatment in Newly Admitted Schizophrenic Patients, Arch Gen Psychiat 25: 404-409, 1971

369. Orlov, P., Kasparian, G., Dimascio, A., Cole, J.O.: Withdrawal of Antiparkinson Drugs, Arch Gen Psychiat 25: 410-412, 1971

370. Ludwig, A.M.: Self-Regulation of the Sensory Environment, Arch Gen Psychiat 25: 413-418, 1971

371. Horowitz, M.S.: Cognitive Response to Stressful Stimuli, Arch Gen Psychiat 25: 419-428, 1971

372. Gaarder, K.: Control of States of Consciousness, Arch Gen Psychiat 25: 436-441, 1971

373. Reiss, D.: Intimacy and Problem Solving, Arch Gen Psychiat 25: 442-255, 1971

374. Clendenin, W.W., Murphy, G.E.: Wrist Cutting, Arch Gen Psychiat 25: 465-469, 1971

375.   Szasz, T.: The Ethics of Addiction, Am J Psychiat 128: 541-546, 1971

376.   Cohen, S.: A Commentary of "The Ethics of Addiction",
        Am J Psychiat 128: 547-550, 1971

377.   Hughes, P.H., Crawford, G.A., Barker, N.W., Schumann, S., Jaffe, J.H.:
        The Social Structure of a Heroin Copping Community,
        Am J Psychiat 128: 551-558, 1971

378.   Gordon, R.E.: Psychiatric Screening Through Multiphasic Health Testing,
        Am J Psychiat 128: 559-563, 1971

379.   Henry, G.M., Wiengartner, H., Murphy, D.L.: Idiosyncratic Patterns of
        Learning and Word Association During Mania,
        Am J Psychiat 128: 564-574, 1971

380.   Reifler, C.B., Howard, J., Lipton, M.A., Liptzin, M.B., Widman, D.E.:
        Pornography: An Experimental Study of Effects,
        Am J Psychiat 128: 575-582, 1971

381.   Rothenberg, E.W., Gody, H., Sands, R.M.: The Vicissitudes of the Adop-
        tion Process, Am J Psychiat 128: 590-597, 1971

382.   Shader, R., Ebert, M.H., Harmantz, J.S.: Langner's Psychiatric Impair-
        ment Scale, Am J Psychiat 128: 596-601, 1971

383.   Bhattacharyya, D.D., Singh, R.: Behavior Therapy of Hysterical Fits,
        Am J Psychiat 128: 602-606, 1971

384.   Polak, P., Laycob, L.: Rapid Tranquilization,
        Am J Psychiat 128: 640-643, 1971

385.   Tec, L.: The Staccato Syndrome, Am J Psychiat 128: 247-648, 1971

386.   Beigel, A., Murphy, D.L.: Assessing Clinical Characteristics of the Manic
        State, Am J Psychiat 128: 688-694, 1971

387.   Bergman, R.L.: Navajo Peyote Use: Its Apparent Safety,
        Am J Psychiat 128: 695-699, 1971

388.   Stein, S.P., Charles, E.: Emotional Factors in Juvenile Diabetes Mellitus,
        Am J Psychiat 128: 700-704, 1971

389.   Glass, G.S., Heninger G.R., Lansky, M., Talan, K.: Psychiatric
        Emergency Related to the Menstrual Cycle,
        Am J Psychiat 128: 705-711, 1971

390.   Khan, A.U.: "Mama's Boy" Syndrome, Am J Psychiat 128: 712-717, 1971

391.   Sifneos, P.: Changes in Patient's Motivation for Psychotherapy,
        Am J Psychiat 128: 718-721, 1971

392.   Mora, G.: 1971 Anniversaries, Am J Psychiat 128: 728-734, 1971

393.   Dupont, R.L., Ryder, R.G., Grunebaum, H.U.: An Unexpected Result
        of Psychosis in Marriage, Am J Psychiat 128: 735-739, 1971

394. Grunebaum, H.U., Abernethy, V.D., Rofman, E.S., Weiss, J.L.: The
      Family Planning Attitudes, Practices and Motivations of Mental Patients,
      Am J Psychiat 128: 740-744, 1971

395. Martin, P.A.: Dynamic Considerations of the Hysterical Psychosis,
      Am J Psychiat 128: 745-748, 1971

396. Biele, A.M.: Unwanted Pregnancy: Symptom of Depressive Practice,
      Am J Psychiat 128: 748-754, 1971

397. Babikian, H.M., Goldman, A.: A Study in Teen-Age Pregnancy,
      Am J Psychiat 128: 755-760, 1971

398. Sullivan, P.R.: Learning Theories and Supportive Psychotherapy,
      Am J Psychiat 128: 763-766, 1971

399. Muller, D.J.: The Advantage of the Psychiatric Triage Unit,
      Am J Psychiat 128: 771-774, 1971

400. Campbell, A.M.G., Evans, M., Thomson, J.L.G., Williams, M.J.:
      Cerebral Atrophy in Young Cannabis Smokers, Lancet II: 1219-1224, 1971

401. Beck, A.T.: Role of Fantasies in Psychotherapy and Psychopathology,
      J Nerv Ment Dis 150: 3-17, 1970

402. Bruch, H.: Psychotherapy in Primary Anorexia Nervosa,
      J Nerv Ment Dis 150: 51-67, 1970

403. Freedman, N., Cutler, R., Engelhardt, D.M., Margolis, R.: On the
      Modification of Paranoid Symptomatology,
      J Nerv Ment Dis 150: 68-76, 1970

404. Karp, S.A., Kissin, B., Hustnyer, F.E.: Field Dependence as a Predictor
      of Alcoholic Therapy Dropouts, J Nerv Ment Dis 150: 77-83, 1970

405. Meyer, R.E., DiMascio, A., Stifler, L.: Personality Differences in the
      Response to Stimulant Drugs Administered During a Sleep-Deprived State,
      J Nerv Ment Dis 150:91-101, 1970

406. Howard, K., Rickels, K., Mock, J.E., Lipman, R.S., Covi, L., Baum,
      N.C.: Therapeutic Style and Attribution Rate from Psychiatric Drug
      Treatment, J Nerv Ment Dis 150: 102-110, 1970

407. Faillace, L.A., Snyder, S.H., Weingartner, H.: DOM: Clinical Evaluation
      of a Hallucinogenic Drug, J Nerv Ment Dis 150: 119-126, 1970

408. Pokorney, A.D., Mefferd, R.B., Stevens, G.: Nailfold Capillary Plexes,
      J Nerv Ment Dis 150: 146-154, 1970

409. Evans, F.J., Gustafson, L.A., O'Connell, D.N., Orne, M.T., Shor, R.E.:
      Verbally Induced Behavioral Responses During Sleep,
      J Nerv Ment Dis 150: 171-187, 1970

410. Starker, S., Goodenough, D.R.: Effects of Sleep State and Method of
      Awakening Upon TAT Production at Arousal,
      J Nerv Ment Dis 150: 188-194, 1970

411. Castaldo, V., Shevrin, H.: Different Effect of an Auditory Stimulus as a
      Function of REM and NREM Sleep, J Nerv Ment Dis 150: 195-200, 1970

412. Wadeson, H.S., Bunney, W.E.: Manic-Depressive Art,
      J Nerv Ment Dis 150: 215-231, 1970

413. Dudek, S.Z.: The Artist as Person, J Nerv Ment Dis 150: 232-241, 1970

414. Mark, V.H., Barry, McLardy, T., Ervin, F.: The Destruction of Both
      Anterior Thalamic Nuclei in a Patient with Intractable Agitated Depression,
      J Nerv Ment Dis 150: 266-272, 1970

415. Horowitz, M.J., Cohen, F.M., Skolnikoff, A.Z., Saunders, F.A.: Psycho-
      motor Epilepsy: Rehabilitation After Surgical Treatment,
      J Nerv Ment Dis 150: 273-290, 1970

416. Stinnett, J.L., Hollander, M.H.: Compulsive Self-Mutilation,
      J Nerv Ment Dis 150: 371-375, 1970

417. Emde, R.N., Metcalf, D.R.: An Electroencephalographic Study of
      Behavioral REM States in the Human Newborn,
      J Nerv Ment Dis 150: 376-385, 1970

418. Ferholt, J.B., Stone, W.N.: Severe Delirium After Abrupt Withdrawal of
      Thiothixene in a Chronic Schizophrenic Patient,
      J Nerv Ment Dis 150: 400-403, 1970

419. Silber, A.: An Addendum to the Technique of Psychotherapy With Alcoholics,
      J Nerv Ment Dis 150: 423-437, 1970

420. Dupont, R.L.: The Imposter and His Mother,
      J Nerv Ment Dis 150: 444-448, 1970

421. Small, J.G., Small, I.F., Perez, H.C., Sharpley, P.: EEG and Neuro-
      physiological Studies of Electrically Induced Seizures,
      J Nerv Ment Dis 150: 479-489, 1970

422. McNeil, T.F., Wiegerink, R., Dozier, J.E.: Pregnancy and Birth Com-
      plications in the Births of Seriously, Moderately and Mildly Behaviorally
      Disturbed Children, J Nerv Ment Dis 150: 24-34, 1970

423. Huffer, V., Levin, L., Aronson, H.: Oral Contraceptives, Depression and
      Frigidity, J Nerv Ment Dis 151: 35-41, 1970

424. Levene, H.I., Rigney, F.J.: Law, Preventive Psychiatry, and Therapeutic
      Abortion, J Nerv Ment Dis 151: 60-68, 1970

425. Reich, T., Winokur, G.: Postpartum Psychoses in Patients with Manic-
      Depressive Disease, J Nerv Ment Dis 151: 60-68, 1970

426. Goldstein, H.S., Paedes, H., Small, A.M., Steinberg, M.D.:
      Psychological Differentiation and Specificity of Response,
      J Nerv Ment Dis 151: 97-103, 1970

427. Walker, H.A., Birch, H.G.: Neurointegrative Deficiency in Schizophrenic
      Children, J Nerv Ment Dis 151: 104-113, 1970

428. Fargalla, F.F., Fluch, F.F.: Studies of Mineral Metabolism in Mental
      Depression, J Nerv Ment Dis 151: 120-129, 1970

429. Koulack, D.: Effects of Thirst on Sleep, J Nerv Ment Dis 151: 143-145, 1970

430. Rosenthal, S.H., Wolfsohn, N.L.: Electrosleep,
      J Nerv Ment Dis 151: 146-151, 1970

431. Cooper, L.: Empathy: A Developmental Model,
      J Nerv Ment Dis 151: 169-178, 1970

432. Shanfield, S., Tucker, H.J., Harrow, M., Detre, T.: The Schizophrenic
      Patient and Depressive Symptomatology, J Nerv Ment Dis 151: 203-210, 1970

433. Lynch, J.J.: Psychopathology and the Development of Social Attachment,
      J Nerv Ment Dis 151: 231-244, 1970

434. Cleghorn, J.M., Peterfy, G., Pinter, E.J., Pattlee, C.J.: Verbal
      Anxiety and the Beta Adrenergic Receptors: A Facilitating Mechanism?,
      J Nerv Ment Dis 151: 266-272, 1970

435. Johnson, G., Maccario, M., Gershon, S., Korein, J.: The Effects of
      Lithium on the EEG, Behavior, and Serum Electrolytes,
      J Nerv Ment Dis 151: 273-279, 1970

436. Weitzman, E.L., Shamoian, C.A., Golosow, N.: Identity Diffusion and
      the Transsexual Resolution, J Nerv Ment Dis 151: 295-302, 1970

437. Mitchell, K.M., Berenson, B.G.: Differential Use of Confrontation by
      High and Low Facilitative Therapists, J Nerv Ment Dis 151: 303-309, 1970

438. Appelbaum, S.A., Coyne, L., Siegal, R.S.: Routes to Change in IQ During
      and After Long Term Psychotherapy, J Nerv Ment Dis 151: 310-315, 1970

439. Walker, H.A., Birch, H.G.: Lateral Preference and Right-Left Awareness,
      J Nerv Ment Dis 151: 341-351, 1970

440. Hilburn, W.B.: Dermatoglyphic Findings on a Group of Psychotic Children,
      J Nerv Ment Dis 151: 352-358, 1970

441. Kupfer, D.J., Wyatt, R.J., Snyder, F.: Comparison Between EEG and
      Systematic Nursing Observations of Sleep in Psychiatric Patients,
      J Nerv Ment Dis 151: 361-368, 1970

442. Arkin, A.M., Toth, M.F., Baker, J., Hastey, J.M.: The Frequency of
      Sleep Talking in the Laboratory Among Chronic Sleep Talkers and Good
      Dream Recallers, J Nerv Ment Dis 151: 369-374, 1970

443. Arkin, A.M., Toth, M.F., Baker, J., Hastey, J.M.: The Degree of Con-
      cordance Between the Content of Sleep Talking and Mentation Recalled in
      Wakefulness, J Nerv Ment Dis 151: 375-393, 1970

444. Krippner, S., Ullman, M.: Telepathy and Dreams,
      J Nerv Ment Dis 151: 394-403, 1970

445. Raphling, D.L.: Dreams and Suicide Attempts, J Nerv Ment Dis 151:
      404-410, 1970

446. Hirsch, S.J., Keniston, K.: Psychosocial Issues in Talented College Dropouts, Psychiatry 33: 1-20, 1970

447. Rosenberg, S.D.: Hospital Culture as Collective Defense, Psychiatry 33: 21-35, 1970

448. Steinfeld, G.J.: Parallels Between the Pathological Family and the Mental Hospital, Psychiatry 33: 36-55, 1970

449. Rioch, M.J.: The Work of Wilfred Bion on Groups, Psychiatry 33 : 56-66, 1970

450. McGlothlin, W.H., Arnold, D.O., Rowan, P.K.: Marijuana Use Among Adults, Psychiatry 33: 433-443, 1970

451. Parkes, C.M.: The First Year of Bereavement, Psychiatry 33: 444-467, 1970

452. Rabkin, L.Y.: Parties and Cultural Values: A Kibbutz Example, Psychiatry 33: 482-493, 1970

453. Olivarius, B.R., Roder E.: Reversible Psychosis and Dementia in Myxedema, Acta Psychiat Scand 46: 1-13, 1970

454. Christensen, E., Moller, J.E., Faurbye, A.: Neuropathological Investigation of 28 Brains from Patients with Dyskinesia, Acta Psychiat Scand 46: 14-23, 1970

455. Mandelbrote, B.M., Trick, K.L.K.: Social and Clinical Factors in the Outcome of Schizophrenia, Acta Psychiat Scand 46: 24-34, 1970

456. Saunders, M.K., McClelland, H.T.: The Effects of Phenothiazaine Therapy on Lymphocyte Transformation in Schizophrenia, Acta Psychiat Scand 46: 64-69, 1970

457. Annell, A.L., Gustavson, K.H., Tenstam, J.: Symptomatology in School Boys With Positive Sex Chromatin, Acta Psychiat Scand 46: 71-80, 1970

458. Gottfries, C.G., Gottfries, I., Roos, B.E.: HVA and 5-HIAA in CSF Related to Rated Mental and Motor Impairment in Senile and Presenile Dementia, Acta Psychiat Scand 46: 99-105, 1970

459. Persson, T., Olsson, L., Ortmon, E.: The Kleine-Levin Syndrome, Acta Psychiat Scand 46: 106-110, 1970

460. Kerry, R.J., Liebling, L.I., Owen, G.: Weight Changes in Lithium Responders, Acta Psychiat Scand 46: 238-243, 1970

461. Mangoni, A., Andreoli, V., Cabibbe, F., Mandelli, V.: Body Fluid Distribution in Manic and Depressive Patients Treated with Lithium Carbonate, Acta Psychiat Scand 46: 244-257, 1970

462. Nielsen, J.: Turner's Syndrome in Medical, Neurological and Psychiatric Wards, Acta Psychiat Scand 46: 286-310, 1970

463. Rasmussen, O.S.: Fluphenazine Enanthate in Sesame Oil, A Depot Preparation, Acta Psychiat Scand 46: 311-318, 1970

464. Watt, J.A.G., Askroft, G.W., Daly, R.J., Smythies, J.R.: Some Observations Concerning the "Pink Spot" Reacting Substances in Urine, Acta Psychiat Scand 46: 374-390, 1970

465. Christodoulu, G.N.: Two Cases of Folie a Deux in Husband and Wife, Acta Psychiat Scand 46: 413-419, 1970

466. Ulett, G.A., Akpinar, S., Itil, T.: Hypnosis: Physiological, Pharmacological Reality, Am J Psychiat 128: 799-805, 1972

467. Hertzberg, L.J.: Cancer and the Dying Patient, Am J Psychiat 128: 806-810, 1972

468. Edwards, G.: Murder and Gun Control, Am J Psychiat 128:811-814, 1972

469. Chodoff, P.: Supervision of Psychotherapy with Videotape: Pros and Cons, Am J Psychiat 128: 819-823, 1972

470. Harrow, M., Tucher, G., Himmelhoch, J., Putnam, N.: Schizophrenic "Thought Disorders" After the Acute Phase, Am J Psychiat 128: 824-829, 1972

471. Auerbach, A.H., Luborsky, L., Johnson, M.: Clinicians' Predictions of Outcome of Psychotherapy: A Trial of a Prognostic Index, Am J Psychiat 128: 830-835, 1971

472. Kaufman, E.: A Psychiatrist's Views on Addict Self-Help Programs, Am J Psychiat 128: 846-852, 1972

473. Bowden, C.L., Langenauer, B.J.: Success and Failure in the NARA Addiction Program, Am J Psychiat 128: 853-856, 1971

474. Dupont, R.L.: Heroin Addiction Treatment and Crime Reduction, Am J Psychiat 128: 856-860, 1972

475. Bess, B., Janus, S., Rifkin, A.: Factors in Successful Narcotics Renunciation, Am J Psychiat 128: 861-865, 1972

476. O'Malley J.E., Anderson, W.H., Lazare, A.: Failure of Outpatient Treatment of Drug Abuse, 1. Heroin, Am J Psychiat 128: 865-868, 1972

477. Katz, J.L., Ackman, P., Rothwax, Y., Sacher, E.J., Weiner, H., Hellman, L., Gallagher, T.F.: Psychoendocrine Aspects of Cancer of the Breast, Psychosom Med 32: 1-18, 1970

478. Kasl, S.V., Cobb., J.: Blood Pressure Changes in Men Undergoing Job Loss, Psychosom Med 32: 19-38, 1970

479. Kopell, B.S., Wittner, W.K., Lunde, D., Warrick, G., Edwards, D.: Cortisol Effects on Average Evoked Potential, Alpha-Rhythm, Time Estimation and Two-Flash Fusion Threshold, Psychosom Med 32: 39-49, 1970

480.   Epstein, S. , Coleman, M.: Drive Theories of Schizophrenia,
        Psychosom Med 32: 113-140, 1970

481.   Brown, W. A. , Mueller, P. S.: Psychological Function in Individuals with
        Amyotropic Lateral Sclerosis, Psychosom Med 32: 141-152, 1970

482.   Kales, A. , Tan, T. L. , Kollar, E. J. , Naitoh, P. , Preston, T. A. ,
        Malmstrom, E. J.: Sleep Patterns Following 205 Hours of Sleep Deprivation,
        Psychosom Med 32: 189-200, 1970

483.   Swanson, D. W. , Dinello,F. A.: Follow-up of Patients Starved for Obesity,
        Psychosom Med 32: 209-214, 1970

484.   Kramer, Y., Rosenblum, L. A.: Responses to "Frustration" in One-Year-
        Old Infants, Psychosom Med 32: 243-257, 1970

485.   Zuger, B.: Gender Role Determination, Psychosom Med 32: 449-467, 1970

486.   Jacobs, M. A. , Knapp, P. H. , Rosenthal, S. , Haskell, D.: Psychological
        Aspects of Cigarette Smoking in Men, Psychosom Med 32: 469-485, 1970

487.   Klatskin, E. H. , Eron, L. D.: Projective Test Content During Pregnancy
        and Postpartum Adjustment, Psychosom Med 32: 487-493, 1970

488.   Kopell, B. S. , Wittner, W. K. , Lunde, D. , Warrick, G. , Edwards, D.:
        Influence of Triiodothyronine on Selective Attention in Man as Measured
        by the Visual AEP, Psychosom Med 32: 495-502, 1970

489.   Liljefors, J. , Rahe, R. H. , An Identical Twin Study of Psychosocial
        Factors in Coronary Heart Disease in Sweden,
        Psychosom Med 32: 523-542, 1970

490.   Kernberg, O. F.: Prognostic Considerations Regarding Borderline
        Personality Organization, J Am Psychoanal Assn 19:595-635, 1971

491.   Miller, J. B. M. , Children's Reactions to the Death of a Parent: A Review,
        J Am Psychoanal Assn 19: 697-719, 1971

492.   Freedman, D. A. , Cannady, C. , Robinson, J. S.: Speech and Psychic
        Structure: A Reconsideration of Their Relation,
        J Am Psychoanal Assn 19: 765-779, 1971

493.   Pao, P. N.: Elation, Hypomania and Mania,
        J Am Psychoanal Assn 19: 787-798, 1971

494.   Niederland, W. G.: On Hesperian Depression,
        J Am Psychoanal Assn 19: 799-805, 1971

495.   Barglow, P. , Sadow, L.: Visual Perception: Its Development and Matura-
        tion from Birth to Adulthood, J Am Psychoanal Assn 19: 433-450, 1971

496.   Kernberg, P. F.: The Course of the Analysis of a Narcissistic Personality
        with Hysterical and Compulsive Features,
        J Am Psychoanal Assn 19: 451-471, 1971

497. Sperling, M.: Spider Phobias and Spider Fantasies, J Am Psychoanal Assn 19: 472-498, 1971

498. Langs, R. J.: Day Residues, Recall Residues and Dreams: Reality and the Psyche, J Am Psychoanal Assn 19: 499-523, 1971

499. Siegel, B. L.: The Role of the Mouth in the Search for the Female Phallus, J Am Psychoanal Assn 19: 310-331, 1971

500. Hurn, H. T.: Toward a Paradigm of the Terminal Phase: The Current Status of the Terminal Phase, J Am Psychoanal Assn 19: 332-348, 1971

501. Fisher, C., Byrne, J., Edwards, A., Kahn, E.: A Psychophysiological Study of Nightmares, J Am Psychoanal Assn 18: 747-782, 1970

502. Kernberg, O. F.: A Psychoanalytic Classification of Character Pathology, J Am Psychoanal Assn 18: 800-822, 1970

503. Anthony, E. J.: Two Contrasting Types of Adolescent Depression and Their Treatment, Am J Psychoanal Assn 18:841-859, 1970

504. Silber, A.: Functional Phenomenon: Historical Concept, Contemporary Defense, J Am Psychoanal Assn 18: 519-538, 1970

505. Stern, M. M.: Therapeutic Playback, Self Objectification and the Analytic Process, J Am Psychoanal Assn 18: 562-598, 1970

506. Ross, N.: The Primacy of Genitality in the Light of Ego Psychology, J Am Psychoanal Assn 18: 267-284, 1970

507. Bak, R. C.: Psychoanalysis Today, J Am Psychoanal Assn 18: 3-23, 1970

508. Frosch, J.: Psychoanalytic Consideration of the Psychotic Character, J Am Psychoanal Assn 24-50, 1970

509. Kernberg, O. F.: Factors in the Psychoanalytic Treatment of Narcissistic Personalities, J Am Psychoanal Assn 18 : 51-85, 1970

510. Harrison, S. T.: Is Psychoanalysis "Our Science"?, J Am Psychoanal Assn 18: 125-149, 1970

511. Winokur, M., Bloom, J.: Stability and Variability of Seat Preference in a Therapy Group: Their Relationships to Patient Behavior, Psychiatry 35: 78-88, 1972

512. Weiner, I. B.: Perspectives on the Modern Adolescent, Psychiatry 35: 20-31, 1972

513. Suomi, S. J., Harlow, H. F., McKinney, W. T.: Monkey Psychiatrists, Am J Psychiat 128: 927-938, 1972

514. Gibson, R. W.: Can Mental Health be Included in the Health Maintenance Organization, Am J Psychiat 128: 919-926, 1972

515.   Roth, M.: Human Violence as Viewed from the Psychiatric Clinic,
        Am J Psychiat 128: 1043-1056, 1972

516.   Rosenberg, A.H., McGarry, A.C.: Competency for Trial: The Making of
        an Expert, Am J Psychiat 128: 1092-1096, 1972

517.   Fieve, R.R.: Lithium in Psychiatry, Int J Psychiat 9: 375-412, 1970-71

518.   Caffey, E.M., Hollister, L.E., Kaim, S.C., Pokorney, A.D.: Drug
        Treatment in Psychiatry, Int J Psychiat 9 : 428-471, 1970-71

519.   Freud, S.: The Interpretation of Dreams, Standard Edition, Hogarth
        Press, London, 1953

520.   Grinspoon, L.: Marijuana, Int J Psychiat 9 : 488-516, 1970-71

521.   Dimascio, A., Shader, R.I., eds.: Clinical Handbook of Psychopharmacol-
        ogy, Science House, New York, 1970

The author has taken great pain to thoroughly check the questions and answers. However, in a volume of this size, some ambiguities and possible inaccuracies may appear. Therefore, if in doubt, consult your references.

THE PUBLISHERS

1. C	51. B	101. E	151. B	201. E
2. A	52. A	102. A	152. B	202. C
3. A	53. D	103. D	153. A	203. B
4. D	54. D	104. B	154. D	204. C
5. D	55. E	105. A	155. E	205. C
6. D	56. C	106. C	156. E	206. E
7. E	57. D	107. B	157. C	207. C
8. B	58. A	108. D	158. D	208. C
9. B	59. E	109. D	159. D	209. B
10. A	60. D	110. A	160. A	210. C
11. B	61. A	111. D	161. E	211. A
12. E	62. C	112. D	162. B	212. D
13. B	63. D	113. B	163. B	213. A
14. E	64. B	114. E	164. E	214. B
15. C	65. D	115. C	165. C	215. A
16. A	66. A	116. A	166. D	216. D
17. E	67. A	117. D	167. A	217. E
18. D	68. D	118. D	168. C	218. C
19. B	69. E	119. A	169. B	219. B
20. D	70. B	120. C	170. B	220. A
21. A	71. B	121. C	171. B	221. D
22. C	72. C	122. E	172. A	222. B
23. C	73. E	123. B	173. A	223. B
24. D	74. E	124. D	174. A	224. D
25. B	75. A	125. A	175. B	225. C
26. A	76. B	126. B	176. D	226. A
27. E	77. A	127. B	177. C	227. B
28. B	78. A	128. E	178. B	228. E
29. A	79. E	129. B	179. C	229. C
30. A	80. C	130. E	180. E	230. D
31. D	81. D	131. C	181. D	231. E
32. E	82. C	132. A	182. A	232. A
33. C	83. A	133. E	183. E	233. B
34. C	84. E	134. D	184. B	234. A
35. B	85. B	135. D	185. A	235. E
36. C	86. B	136. A	186. B	236. C
37. B	87. D	137. E	187. C	237. C
38. B	88. C	138. C	188. A	238. B
39. B	89. A	139. A	189. D	239. D
40. A	90. E	140. D	190. D	240. A
41. C	91. C	141. E	191. E	241. A
42. B	92. E	142. E	192. A	242. B
43. C	93. A	143. B	193. D	243. D
44. E	94. B	144. C	194. D	244. D
45. E	95. D	145. A	195. D	245. B
46. C	96. A	146. B	196. B	246. B
47. E	97. A	147. B	197. B	247. B
48. E	98. A	148. B	198. D	248. B
49. C	99. C	149. A	199. E	249. A
50. D	100. D	150. C	200. A	250. C

251.	D	301.	B	351.	E	401.	E	451.	D
252.	E	302.	E	352.	B	402.	C	452.	E
253.	B	303.	D	353.	A	403.	B	453.	C
254.	B	304.	E	354.	B	404.	E	454.	E
255.	D	305.	A	355.	D	405.	A	455.	E
256.	C	306.	E	356.	C	406.	C	456.	E
257.	D	307.	B	357.	D	407.	D	457.	E
258.	A	308.	A	358.	C	408.	A	458.	C
259.	C	309.	E	359.	E	409.	D	459.	D
260.	D	310.	D	360.	A	410.	A	460.	A
261.	C	311.	D	361.	A	411.	B	461.	E
262.	A	312.	A	362.	E	412.	E	462.	B
263.	D	313.	A	363.	A	413.	A	463.	E
264.	D	314.	A	364.	C	414.	A	464.	A
265.	C	315.	C	365.	C	415.	B	465.	D
266.	D	316.	B	366.	A	416.	E	466.	B
267.	E	317.	B	367.	E	417.	D	467.	C
268.	A	318.	D	368.	B	418.	A	468.	D
269.	B	319.	A	369.	D	419.	D	469.	A
270.	E	320.	D	370.	A	420.	A	470.	C
271.	A	321.	A	371.	A	421.	A	471.	A
272.	C	322.	C	372.	C	422.	C	472.	B
273.	D	323.	D	373.	C	423.	D	473.	B
274.	A	324.	E	374.	B	424.	D	474.	E
275.	C	325.	B	375.	A	425.	A	475.	B
276.	A	326.	E	376.	E	426.	C	476.	C
277.	C	327.	D	377.	B	427.	B	477.	D
278.	A	328.	B	378.	C	428.	E	478.	B
279.	A	329.	B	379.	D	429.	D	479.	D
280.	A	330.	C	380.	E	430.	D	480.	A
281.	B	331.	A	381.	D	431.	A	481.	B
282.	A	332.	C	382.	A	432.	D	482.	B
283.	C	333.	E	383.	C	433.	A	483.	D
284.	A	334.	B	384.	E	434.	B	484.	C
285.	A	335.	A	385.	D	435.	C	485.	C
286.	D	336.	B	386.	B	436.	E	486.	D
287.	B	337.	A	387.	A	437.	C	487.	C
288.	B	338.	C	388.	E	438.	E	488.	D
289.	A	339.	D	389.	D	439.	E	489.	B
290.	E	340.	A	390.	B	440.	B	490.	A
291.	D	341.	C	391.	B	441.	D	491.	E
292.	C	342.	B	392.	A	442.	A	492.	A
293.	D	343.	E	393.	D	443.	E	493.	C
294.	C	344.	A	394.	B	444.	C	494.	B
295.	D	345.	D	395.	E	445.	D	495.	E
296.	D	346.	B	396.	A	446.	D	496.	C
297.	A	347.	B	397.	B	447.	A	497.	C
298.	E	348.	C	398.	E	448.	C	498.	E
299.	A	349.	A	399.	D	449.	D	499.	B
300.	E	350.	C	400.	A	450.	A	500.	B

501. E	551. D	601. C	651. E	701. B
502. B	552. D	602. B	652. D	702. C
503. D	553. D	603. B	653. A	703. E
504. B	554. B	604. A	654. A	704. A
505. A	555. D	605. A	655. D	705. B
506. D	556. C	606. E	656. A	706. A
507. A	557. B	607. E	657. C	707. A
508. E	558. C	608. E	658. B	708. A
509. A	559. E	609. E	659. A	709. B
510. E	560. D	610. D	660. E	710. C
511. A	561. E	611. C	661. C	711. D
512. E	562. E	612. C	662. A	712. D
513. E	563. E	613. B	663. A	713. E
514. E	564. A	614. C	664. A	714. A
515. B	565. E	615. A	665. A	715. C
516. A	566. D	616. B	666. C	716. A
517. A	567. E	617. D	667. C	717. A
518. D	568. B	618. E	668. D	718. D
519. C	569. E	619. C	669. C	719. B
520. D	570. B	620. B	670. B	720. A
521. A	571. D	621. D	671. E	721. B
522. D	572. C	622. B	672. A	722. B
523. B	573. A	623. B	673. B	723. E
524. E	574. D	624. B	674. C	724. D
525. C	575. B	625. A	675. D	725. C
526. D	576. B	626. C	676. C	726. B
527. C	577. E	627. A	677. A	727. E
528. C	578. C	628. C	678. B	728. A
529. E	579. A	629. A	679. D	729. D
530. A	580. A	630. E	680. A	730. C
531. A	581. C	631. D	681. C	731. C
532. A	582. D	632. E	682. E	732. D
533. E	583. C	633. E	683. B	733. E
534. A	584. C	634. D	684. B	734. A
535. E	585. E	635. B	685. B	735. B
536. B	586. A	636. C	686. C	736. E
537. C	587. A	637. A	687. A	737. B
538. D	588. E	638. B	688. C	738. A
539. B	589. C	639. A	689. A	739. C
540. D	590. E	640. A	690. D	740. D
541. A	591. A	641. C	691. B	741. D
542. D	592. D	642. C	692. C	742. A
543. E	593. C	643. C	693. D	743. B
544. D	594. B	644. C	694. E	744. D
545. A	595. A	645. B	695. C	745. B
546. A	596. B	646. D	696. B	746. E
547. B	597. B	647. E	697. B	747. C
548. D	598. E	648. A	698. E	748. E
549. A	599. A	649. B	699. A	749. D
550. C	600. D	650. D	700. D	750. D

751.	E	801.	A	851.	B	901.	D	951.	E
752.	D	802.	E	852.	B	902.	B	952.	B
753.	B	803.	A	853.	B	903.	A	953.	A
754.	E	804.	E	854.	B	904.	A	954.	D
755.	C	805.	B	855.	B	905.	D	955.	A
756.	C	806.	A	856.	D	906.	E	956.	B
757.	A	807.	C	857.	A	907.	D	957.	C
758.	A	808.	B	858.	C	908.	B	958.	A
759.	E	809.	B	859.	C	909.	C	959.	C
760.	A	810.	C	860.	E	910.	B	960.	D
761.	A	811.	D	861.	D	911.	E	961.	B
762.	A	812.	D	862.	C	912.	A	962.	A
763.	E	813.	D	863.	B	913.	B	963.	D
764.	A	814.	E	864.	C	914.	E	964.	E
765.	E	815.	E	865.	D	915.	C	965.	A
766.	B	816.	E	866.	D	916.	A	966.	D
767.	D	817.	A	867.	D	917.	E	967.	D
768.	D	818.	B	868.	E	918.	A	968.	C
769.	C	819.	C	869.	D	919.	A	969.	E
770.	B	820.	A	870.	C	920.	B	970.	D
771.	A	821.	C	871.	D	921.	D	971.	D
772.	A	822.	D	872.	D	922.	A	972.	A
773.	E	823.	E	873.	A	923.	C	973.	E
774.	B	824.	B	874.	E	924.	C	974.	E
775.	C	825.	C	875.	B	925.	E	975.	A
776.	A	826.	A	876.	C	926.	A	976.	B
777.	E	827.	B	877.	D	927.	C	977.	E
778.	A	828.	E	878.	E	928.	D	978.	E
779.	A	829.	D	879.	D	929.	A	979.	C
780.	D	830.	A	880.	E	930.	D	980.	A
781.	A	831.	E	881.	D	931.	B	981.	A
782.	D	832.	C	882.	B	932.	A	982.	C
783.	B	833.	D	883.	B	933.	E	983.	E
784.	E	834.	C	884.	A	934.	B	984.	C
785.	E	835.	D	885.	D	935.	A	985.	E
786.	B	836.	B	886.	B	936.	D	986.	B
787.	A	837.	A	887.	A	937.	C	987.	C
788.	D	838.	A	888.	C	938.	D	988.	D
789.	C	839.	D	889.	C	939.	B	989.	B
790.	C	840.	A	890.	E	940.	C	990.	C
791.	D	841.	C	891.	A	941.	E	991.	E
792.	E	842.	A	892.	B	942.	A	992.	D
793.	C	843.	D	893.	B	943.	A	993.	A
794.	C	844.	B	894.	E	944.	E	994.	E
795.	B	845.	A	895.	C	945.	A	995.	C
796.	D	846.	A	896.	E	946.	E	996.	A
797.	E	847.	A	897.	E	947.	A	997.	E
798.	E	848.	B	898.	A	948.	A	998.	E
799.	B	849.	A	899.	C	949.	E	999.	D
800.	A	850.	B	900.	D	950.	D	1000.	C

1001. B	1051. A	1101. D	1151. C
1002. D	1052. A	1102. B	1152. B
1003. A	1053. A	1103. A	1153. E
1004. D	1054. B	1104. E	1154. C
1005. D	1055. B	1105. A	1155. E
1006. D	1056. D	1106. E	1156. D
1007. B	1057. D	1107. A	1157. B
1008. A	1058. C	1108. B	1158. C
1009. C	1059. E	1109. D	1159. D
1010. A	1060. B	1110. B	1160. D
1011. E	1061. B	1111. A	1161. C
1012. A	1062. A	1112. B	1162. A
1013. A	1063. C	1113. C	1163. A
1014. E	1064. D	1114. C	1164. D
1015. E	1065. C	1115. E	1165. B
1016. C	1066. E	1116. E	1166. D
1017. D	1067. D	1117. A	1167. B
1018. B	1068. C	1118. A	1168. C
1019. D	1069. A	1119. C	1169. A
1020. C	1070. D	1120. B	1170. D
1021. E	1071. B	1121. E	1171. D
1022. C	1072. B	1122. C	1172. B
1023. A	1073. A	1123. D	1173. E
1024. A	1074. E	1124. A	1174. C
1025. B	1075. C	1125. B	1175. B
1026. B	1076. A	1126. B	1176. C
1027. D	1077. B	1127. D	1177. A
1028. E	1078. C	1128. D	1178. D
1029. C	1079. E	1129. E	1179. A
1030. D	1080. A	1130. C	1180. D
1031. B	1081. B	1131. A	1181. **D**
1032. A	1082. A	1132. C	1182. E
1033. D	1083. E	1133. D	1183. D
1034. D	1084. D	1134. E	1184. D
1035. D	1085. E	1135. C	1185. B
1036. E	1086. D	1136. E	1186. A
1037. A	1087. E	1137. E	1187. E
1038. C	1088. A	1138. D	1188. A
1039. C	1089. B	1139. D	1189. E
1040. E	1090. E	1140. E	1190. E
1041. A	1091. D	1141. B	1191. A
1042. B	1092. C	1142. E	1192. D
1043. A	1093. B	1143. A	1193. E
1044. A	1094. D	1144. C	1194. A
1045. D	1095. C	1145. C	1195. B
1046. A	1096. A	1146. A	1196. E
1047. E	1097. D	1147. C	1197. E
1048. B	1098. E	1148. C	1198. A
1049. E	1099. B	1149. A	1199. E
1050. D	1100. D	1150. D	1200. E

OTHER BOOKS AVAILABLE

I T E M S	Code	Unit Price	I T E M S	Code	Unit Price
MEDICAL EXAM REVIEW BOOKS			**STATE BOARD REVIEW BOOKS**		
Vol. 1 Comprehensive	101	$12.00	Med. State Brd. Rev. - Basic Sciences	411	$9.00
Vol. 2 Clinical Medicine	102	7.50	Med. State Brd. Rev. -Clinical Sciences	412	9.00
Vol. 2A Txtbk. Study Guide of Int. Med.	123	7.50	Cardiopulmonary Techn. Exam. Rev. - Vol.1	473	7.50
Vol. 2B Txtbk. Study Guide of Int. Med.	130	7.50	Cytology Exam. Review Book - Vol. 1	454	7.50
Vol. 3 Basic Sciences	103	7.50	Dental Exam. Review Book - Vol. 1	431	7.50
Vol. 4 Obstetrics - Gynecology	104	7.50	Dental Exam. Review Book - Vol. 2	432	7.50
Vol. 4A Textbk. Study Guide of Gynecology	152	7.50	Dental Exam. Review Book - Vol. 3	433	7.50
Vol. 5 Surgery	105	7.50	Dental Hygiene Exam. Review - Vol. 1	461	7.50
Vol. 5A Textbk. Study Guide of Surgery	150	7.50	Emergency Med. Techn. Exam. Rev. - Vol.1	465	7.50
Vol. 6 Public Health & Prev. Medicine	106	7.50	Emergency Med. Techn. Exam. Rev. - Vol.2	466	7.50
Vol. 8 Psychiatry & Neurology	108	7.50	Immunology Exam. Review Book - Vol. 1	424	7.50
Vol.11 Pediatrics	111	7.50	Inhalation Therapy Exam. Review - Vol. 1	471	7.50
Vol.12 Anesthesiology	112	7.50	Inhalation Therapy Exam. Review - Vol. 2	344	7.50
Vol.13 Orthopaedics	113	10.00	Laboratory Asst. Exam. Rev. Bk. - Vol. 1	455	7.50
Vol.14 Urology	114	10.00	Medical Librarian Exam. Rev. Bk. - Vol. 1	495	7.50
Vol.15 Ophthalmology	115	10.00	Medical Record Library Science - Vol. 1	496	7.50
Vol.16 Otolaryngology	116	10.00	Medical Techn. Exam. Review - Vol. 1	451	7.50
Vol.17 Radiology	117	10.00	Medical Techn. Exam. Review - Vol. 2	452	7.50
Vol.18 Thoracic Surgery	118	10.00	Occupational Therapy Exam. Rev. - Vol.1	475	7.50
Vol.19 Neurological Surgery	119	15.00	Optometry Exam. Review	469	10.00
Vol.20 Physical Medicine	128	10.00	Pharmacy Exam. Review Book - Vol. 1	421	7.50
Vol.21 Dermatology	127	10.00	Physical Therapy Exam. Review - Vol. 1	481	7.50
Vol.22 Gastroenterology	141	10.00	Physical Therapy Exam. Review - Vol. 2	482	7.50
Vol.23 Child Psychiatry	126	10.00	X-Ray Technology Exam. Rev. - Vol. 1	441	7.50
Vol.24 Pulmonary Diseases	143	10.00	X-Ray Technology Exam. Rev. - Vol. 2	442	7.50
Vol.25 Nuclear Medicine	133	10.00	X-Ray Technology Exam. Rev. - Vol. 3	443	7.50
Vol.26 Allergy	132	10.00	**NURSING EXAM REVIEW BOOKS**		
Vol.27 Plastic Surgery	129	10.00	Vol. 1 Medical-Surgical Nursing	501	4.50
Vol.28 Cardiovascular Diseases	138	10.00	Vol. 2 Psychiatric-Mental Health Nursing	502	4.50
Vol.29 Oncology	146	10.00	Vol. 3 Maternal-Child Health Nursing	503	4.50
ECFMG Exam Review - Part One	120	7.50	Vol. 4 Basic Sciences	504	4.50
ECFMG Exam Review - Part Two	121	7.50	Vol. 5 Anatomy and Physiology	505	4.50
BASIC SCIENCE REVIEW BOOKS			Vol. 6 Pharmacology	506	4.50
Anatomy Review	201	7.00	Vol. 7 Microbiology	507	4.50
Biochemistry Review	202	7.00	Vol. 8 Nutrition & Diet Therapy	508	4.50
Digestive System Basic Sciences	215	7.00	Vol. 9 Community Health	509	4.50
Heart & Vascular Systems Basic Sciences	212	7.00	Vol.10 History & Law of Nursing	510	4.50
Microbiology Review	203	7.00	Vol.11 Fundamentals of Nursing	511	4.50
Nervous System Basic Sciences	210	7.00	Practical Nursing Examination Rev.- Vol.1	711	4.50
Pathology Review	204	7.00	**CASE STUDY BOOKS**		
Pharmacology Review	205	7.00	Allergy Case Studies	027	10.00
Physiology Review	206	7.00	Cardiology Case Studies	001	10.00
Respiratory System Basic Sciences	213	7.00	Chest Diseases Case Studies	012	10.00
Urinary System B.Sci.	214	7.00	Child Psychiatry Case Studies	029	10.00
Anatomy Textbook Study Guide	124	7.00	Cutaneous Medicine Case Studies	014	7.50
Histology Textbook Study Guide	151	7.00	ECG Case Studies	003	7.50
Medical Physiology Textbk. Study Guide	155	7.00	Endocrinology Case Studies	008	10.00
SPECIALTY BOARD REVIEW BOOKS			Gastroenterology Case Studies	004	10.00
Dermatology Specialty Board Review	311	10.00	Hematology Case Studies	020	10.00
Family Practice Specialty Board Review	309	10.00	Infectious Diseases Case Studies	011	7.50
Internal Medicine Specialty Board Review	303	10.00	Neurology Case Studies	006	10.00
Neurology Specialty Board Review	306	10.00	Orthopedic Surgery Case Studies	030	10.00
Obstetrics-Gynecology Spec. Bd. Review	304	10.00	Otolaryngology Case Studies	021	10.00
Pathology Specialty Board Review	305	10.00	Pediatric Hematology Case Studies	018	10.00
Pediatrics Specialty Board Review	301	10.00	Pediatric Oculo-Neural Dis. Case Studies	023	10.00
Psychiatry Specialty Board Review	312	10.00	Respiratory Care Case Studies	019	7.50
Surgery Specialty Board Review	302	10.00	Urology Case Studies	017	10.00
The Otolaryngology Boards	313	10.00	**MEDICAL OUTLINE SERIES**		
The Psychiatry Boards	307	8.00	Cancer Chemotherapy	631	10.00
			Child Psychiatry	613	10.00

Prices subject to change.

OTHER BOOKS AVAILABLE

ITEMS	Code	Unit Price	ITEMS	Code	Unit Price
MEDICAL OUTLINE SERIES (Cont'd.)			Institutional Laundry Journal Articles	789	$8.00
Endocrinology	614	$10.00	Lithium & Psychiatry Journal Articles	520	15.00
Histology	662	8.00	Psychosomatic Medicine Current J. Art.	788	12.00
Otolaryngology	661	8.00	Outpatient Services Journal Articles, 2nd Ed.	797	10.00
Psychiatry	621	8.00	Outpatient Services Journal Articles, *1st Ed.*	794	8.00
Urology	611	8.00	Selected Papers in Inhalation Therapy	523	10.00
SELF-ASSESSMENT BOOKS			**TYPIST HANDBOOKS**		
Self-Assess. Cur. Knldge - Biochemistry	266	7.50	Medical Typist's Guide for Hx & Phys.	976	4.50
S.A.C.K. in Cardiovascular Diseases	275	10.00	Radiology Typist Handbook	981	4.50
S.A.C.K. in Diagnostic Radiology	278	10.00	Surgical Typist Handbook	991	4.50
S.A.C.K. in Family Practice	261	10.00	Transcribers Guide to Med. Terminology	973	4.50
S.A.C.K. in Infectious Diseases	263	10.00	**ESSAY Q. & A. REVIEW BOOKS**		
S.A.C.K. in Internal Medicine	257	10.00	Blood Banking Principles Rev.	339	8.00
S.A.C.K. in Neurology	254	10.00	Cardiology Review	337	10.00
S.A.C.K. for Nurse Anesthetist	715	7.50	Colon & Rectal Surg. Cont. Ed. Rev.	338	10.00
S.A.C.K. in Obstet./Gynecology	260	10.00	Neurology Review	345	10.00
S.A.C.K. in O.R. Techn.	474	7.50	Obstet. Nursing Cont. Ed. Rev.	350	5.00
S.A.C.K. in Otolaryngology	270	10.00	Ophthalmology Review	347	10.00
S.A.C.K. in Pathology	253	10.00	Orthopedics Review	349	10.00
S.A.C.K. in Pediatrics	256	10.00	Psychiatry Cont. Ed. Rev.	352	10.00
S.A.C.K. in Psychiatry	252	10.00	Psych./Mental Hlth. Nursing Cont. Ed. Rev.	351	5.00
S.A.C.K. in Pulmonary Diseases	271	10.00	**OTHER BOOKS**		
S.A.C.K. in Rheumatology	258	10.00	Acid Base Homeostasis	601	4.00
S.A.C.K. in Surgery	250	10.00	Allergy Annual Review	325	12.00
S.A.C.K. in Surgery for Family Physicians	259	10.00	Bailey & Love's Short Practice of Surgery	900	20.00
S.A.C.K. in Urology	251	10.00	Benign & Malignant Bladder Tumors	932	15.00
S.A.C.K. in X-Ray Tech.	274	7.50	Blood Groups	860	2.50
MEDICAL HANDBOOKS			Clinical Diagnostic Pearls	730	4.50
E.N.T. Emergencies	639	8.00	Concentrations of Solutions	602	3.00
Medical Emergencies	635	8.00	Critical Care Manual	983	10.00
Neurology	604	8.00	Cryogenics in Surgery	754	24.00
Obstetrical Emergencies	634	8.00	Diagnosis & Treatment of Breast Lesions	748	15.00
Ophthalmologic Emergencies	633	8.00	Emergency Care Manual	984	7.50
Pediatric Anesthesia	637	8.00	English-Spanish Guide for Med. Personnel	721	2.50
Pediatric Neurology	636	10.00	Fundamental Orthopedics	603	4.50
PRACTICAL POINTS BOOKS			Guide to Medical Reports	962	4.50
In Anesthesiology	700	10.00	Human Anatomical Terminology	982	3.00
In Gastroenterology	733	7.00	Illustrated Laboratory Techniques	919	10.00
In Pediatrics	702	10.00	Introduction to Acupuncture	753	5.00
PRACTITIONERS GUIDES			Introduction to Blood Banking	975	8.00
OB-Gynecology Disorders	704	10.00	Introduction to the Clinical History	729	3.00
Ophthalmologic Disorders	703	10.00	Lab. Diagnosis of Inf. Dis.	965	7.50
JOURNAL ARTICLE COMPILATIONS			Math for Med Techs	964	7.00
Ambulance Service Journal Articles	517	10.00	Multilingual Guide for Medical Personnel	961	2.50
Blood Banking & Immunohemat. Jour. Art.	798	10.00	Neoplasms of the Gastrointestinal Tract	736	20.00
Emergency Room Journal Articles	795	8.00	Neurophysiology Study Guide	600	7.00
Hodgkin's Disease Journal Articles	515	12.00	Nursing & the Nephrology Patient	376	5.00
Hosp. & Inst. Eng. & Maintenance J. Art.	793	8.00	Outpatient Hemorrhoidectomy Lig. Tech.	752	12.50
Hosp. Electronic Data Process. J. Art.	791	8.00	Profiles in Surgery, Gynec. & Obstetrics	963	5.00
Hosp. Pharmacy Journal Articles	799	10.00	Radiological Physics Exam. Review	486	10.00
Hosp. Security & Safety Journal Articles	796	8.00	Skin, Heredity & Malignant Neoplasms	744	20.00
Human Cytomegalovirus Journal Articles	522	15.00	Testicular Tumors	743	20.00
Immunosuppressive Therapy Journal Art.	526	20.00	Tissue Adhesives in Surgery	756	24.00
			Understanding Hematology	977	8.00

Prices subject to change.